BREAK FREE FROM PAIN

KIRSTY BORTOFT

DISCLAIMER

All information obtained from Kirsty Bortoft, said or written by her, is to be taken as advisory in nature. Kirsty Bortoft, a Mindset Coach and founder of the Freedom Alignment Method will not be financially, legally or personally liable for any action taken based upon her advice. The reader takes full responsibility for the way they utilise and exercise information in this book.

ACKNOWLEDGMENT

Dedicated to my three amazing sons Ethan, Toby and Aspen Bortoft. To my parents, Michael and Fiona Bortoft, who have been integral to my path unfolding the way it has. To Stuart Clark who is my world. Lastly, to whom I am eternally grateful, my spiritual teacher Maharishi Krishnananda Ishaya.

THANK YOU

Thank you to each and every client and student that I have ever had the pleasure to work with. I want to say a huge thank you to Carolyn Sykes for your unwavering support and guidance. Thank you to Purya Ishaya for editing this book and being my partner in crime when teaching The Bright Path Ascension Meditation. Also, thank you to Lesley Hodgson for help with the final read through. To Prema Lee Gurreri, for being my solid mentor, coach and Jyotish Teacher. To Lizzie Hannington for being a Rockstar, for her patience and ability to not take any of this journey seriously. Finally, thank you to Stuart Clark, who believes in me beyond words, inspires me each and every day and loves me unconditionally. You are the person who gets me over the finish line each and every time. I feel so blessed to have you in my life. Thank you.

INDEX

FOREWORD

I first met Kirsty, an Ishaya monk, when she came to teach a meditation weekend at my home. Well, that was the first official meeting anyway. I had glimpsed her at another meditation course a year earlier. There were more than 100 people in attendance and apart from the teacher, who glowed with another-worldly light, Kirsty was the only person who struck me and remained in my memory, even though we had never met or spoken. It was her presence that imprinted upon me.

When she arrived at my home comm moments later, I instantly felt I had met a kindred spirit. What struck me most about her was her kindness, her ease in talking to anyone - and making them feel welcome, and of course that magnetic presence.

Immediately following the weekend, we became the firmest of friends, catching up on video calls multiple times per week. We have shared everything over the last 24 months - successes and challenges. I can be my most authentic self when talking to her, and that is a rare thing in today's world!

I had the privilege and honour of assisting her in putting her story down on paper for the book you hold in your hands. I was truly blown away by what this human angel has endured and overcome in her life and the sheer determination to uplift humanity and turn any situation into a positive, not only for herself, but for all of us.

You don't, as yet, realise what value you hold in your hands. I strongly urge you to engage the practices she shares here for your own transformation - and who knows - maybe one day someone will be writing you a foreword like this.

I'm going to 'borrow' a direct quote from Kirsty which she so kindly said about me, but I wholeheartedly cannot think of another human being alive that this applies to more: 'The world needs more Kirsty Bortoft'.

Carolyn Sykes, Acupuncturist & Meditation coach and author of Choose Life.

TESTIMONIALS

CAROL, 56, Scarborough, UK

Almost all of my life I had known chronic, debilitating pain, fatigue, and digestive issues and had used every medication, alternative therapy, therapeutic activity, diet and food supplement that I had researched and could access. Whilst some of these approaches were beneficial, they just helped with symptoms and I got by.... just, (though not always, there were many times that I struggled to cope). Five years ago, I struggled to walk as far as the end of my road, I needed to use crutches and considered getting a mobility scooter.

I was always on a constant mission to make things easier for myself so that I could maintain my work and family responsibilities. Sometimes that was too much of a struggle and I succumbed to enforced rest. I completely changed my life and lifestyle, always chasing a cure, always striving towards a pain-free life.

I had begun to accept that living with pain and virtually housebound was my lot and I had just got to make the best of it. I had developed a positive attitude and always made sure I did something I enjoyed every day, even if that was just looking at the view out of my window or looking at pretty images on Pinterest.

I was sceptical when I first heard about Kirsty, after all, I thought I had tried everything. I had seen her promotional material and dismissed it, thinking a cure for this was impossible. Then a friend introduced me to her and told me that she had been cured of fibromyalgia. Cured.

So, I met with her over coffee for an initial consultation to see if she could work with me. After that first meeting, I felt hope, and I thought, 'what do I have to lose?' Pain... that's what... and with that trust, I started to learn the Freedom Alignment Method (F.A.M).

It was tough, I had to dive deep into my internal world and root out the causes of the illness. I experienced more intense pain as a part of the process but noticed how I was changing and how, bit by bit, I was clearing all the complex emotional charge that had fed the disease. Kirsty supported me all the way with insight and expertise. I felt held, understood, and reassured that I could get better.

Today, almost 18 months on, I am living a pain-free life. I'm so grateful to enjoy my health. I'm able to live my life without the restrictions that fibromyalgia brings and I'm enjoying life and thriving. I can make plans and get out and about, I am rebuilding a healthy social life and my work life is benefiting too. I have more time and energy to devote to my business. It's a new and exciting chapter because now I believe that so much more is possible for me. Kirsty Bortoft transforms lives – fact.

Leanne, 52, Australia

After having fibromyalgia for five years, I believed it was just something I was going to have to live with for the rest of my life. A friend gave me Kirsty's details and I knew before the end of my free consultation that I would finally be pain free. Kirsty's confidence, commitment and 'it's only going one way - up' attitude was infectious. I have loved every session. She is a beautiful, compassionate and caring woman and I feel so grateful to her. Two months after we started working together and I can now tie my shoes on my own, I am exercising again, I am starting a new business and my relationships are flourishing. My fibromyalgia and osteoarthritis are gone, and for the first time in a very long time, I feel excited about my life.

Laura, 40, UK

When I first met Kirsty, I was in so much pain. I had ruptured a disc in my back in a surfing accident and it was pressing on my spinal nerve. It was causing constant sciatic pain and cramps in my legs. I was waiting for an operation to fix the disc that would involve several months of recovery. All my usual activities were on hold. Even walking, showering or washing up were excruciating. Kirsty assured me that she could get me pain free. What followed was miraculous. Five weeks before I was due to have my operation, I was completely pain free and I am still pain free and fully active one year later.

<u>Lynne, 56, UK</u>

I had been suffering with osteoarthritis and it had reached such a point that I was considering a hip replacement. I heard about Kirsty and I thought I didn't have anything to lose, although I have to say that I was rather sceptical at first. In just four sessions I had gone from a 10 on the pain score, being hardly able to walk, to a zero! I'm amazed and so grateful. She is literally the Goddess who removes pain.

<u>Linzi, 38, Isle of Man</u>

I was suffering from extreme fatigue and constant pain. I couldn't imagine being without pain. I couldn't walk without being in agony. I could not sleep. I could not work and I was so tired and depressed. I felt like I was old beyond my years. Kirsty is inspiring and confident. She makes you believe that it is going to work. She inspires you to realise that you are the person making it work. This programme treats the cause, not the symptoms. Kirsty gently coaches you into the new you. She teaches you to live in the present, go with the flow, step away and embrace a pain free, happy future.

Lizzie, 40, UK

I had experienced tricky mental health for 25 years. I had my first of several mental breakdowns at 16. By the time I reached my late thirties, I was on very high doses of different medications which kept me barely functioning. I was well-aware of what had caused my mental instability, I just couldn't find a way to stop the intrusive, negative thought patterns. I had taken part in several different forms of counselling, psychotherapy, CBT, and mindfulness therapies over the years but nothing lasted for long. It just felt like a sticking plaster, holding all the broken bits together. Seemingly by chance, I was offered an opportunity to join a pilot programme run by Kirsty, and I grabbed it. To say it saved my life is not an understatement. Within two months I was reducing my medication and within four months I was completely medication free and I continue to be so - six months on. I am now working part-time, whilst setting up my own business and finally fully loving and embracing my life. For the first time in 25 years, I love the life I live and the people in it. Most importantly, I finally love myself.

Amelie, 13, UK

I had struggled with being worried for a long time. When I was at primary school, I always felt anxious and worried and I just wanted to be at home with mummy. I would cry and have panic attacks and when I got to year 7 it got a lot worse. When I started working with Kirsty, she made me feel like I was normal. I had had counselling and worked with Child and Adolescent Mental Health Services (CAMHS), but this was the first time I walked away from a session and didn't feel like there was something wrong or broken in me. I loved my sessions with Kirsty. She was fun and really understood me. After six weeks I had the tools to use when I am feeling low or anxious. She taught me how to be confident and how to be brave. I now feel a lot more confident in myself. If I have a wobble, I know she is always there if I need her.

Millie, 14, UK

When I met Kirsty, my mind was controlling me – I had no control over the anxiety I was feeling. Which made me feel stressed and unhappy. Working with Kirsty was an eye-opening experience as it gave me strategies to deal with my stress and anxiety. This made life easier. It gave me a solution to sort out the way I was feeling, which was a huge relief. Talking about everything with someone who wasn't going to judge me, was the best thing. She also gave me a way to solve what I thought were unsolvable problems. Sometimes I found it hard to speak about my feelings but once I got used to it, it wasn't hard any more. Working through this programme has helped me to be happier. Even family and friends have noticed that I have a more positive outlook on things. I stopped making everything so hard. I would definitely recommend working with Kirsty.

I think that every teenager should do it. It has changed my life for the better. I can deal with things when they arise now. I also have a metaphorical tool bag that I will use for life.

Stuart, 45, UK

When I met Kirsty, I wasn't struggling with a particular issue, it was more that I was struggling to stop my emotions getting the better of me. This was initially instigated by a relationship breakdown. The ideals of the Freedom Alignment Method resonated with me instantly. I found myself drawn to the programme and wanted to create a better version of myself. I felt the ideals were already within me and Kirsty found a way to bring these to the surface. I have only just begun this journey, yet feel completely at home with it and find myself growing week by week. I have a much greater awareness of everything! Kirsty and I just clicked, and whilst I appreciate that her task is to be my mindset coach, she must take a huge amount of credit from the way I have developed in this short time. Kirsty has and is continuing to make such an impact on me, I cannot underestimate the strength in what she does, her delivery is fabulous; overwhelming at times. These qualities cannot be taught or learned; she is a real ambassador for the methods. Kirsty has a fantastic ability to impart her understanding to others, especially me. I will be forever indebted to her for what she is doing for me, truly inspiring. I am looking forward to what is next; a world full of endless possibilities!

Jessica, 39, UK

I had suffered chronic pain in my right shoulder for the best part of 20 years. When I was introduced to Kirsty, I was in a particularly bad bout of depression arising from the pain. After a prolonged period of stress at work and my anxiety being through the roof; just getting to my initial appointment was like climbing a mountain, but Kirsty immediately put me at ease and I left feeling so much less of a failure than when I arrived. The best thing that Kirsty has done for me is to show me that I need to look after myself first. If I look after myself, then the rest will naturally follow. There are so many successes that I don't really know where to start; I think first and foremost though has to be pain relief. I am now, probably 90 per cent of the time, completely shoulder pain free. Kirsty has helped me to listen to my body so that, if the shoulder pain is creeping on, I know what is causing it and how to nip it in the bud. Other significant successes include improved mood, diminished anxiety and I'm generally so much happier. If I have a wobble I can reach out to Kirsty and she is never long in replying. With Kirsty's help and support I am about to embark on the next exciting chapter of my journey.

Michelle, 52, UK

When I first met Kirsty, I had just been going through the motions of everyday life for quite a number of years; painting a smile on my face but feeling so empty inside. I'd been carrying years and years of baggage which I didn't realise was actually affecting me and the people around me. I soon realised that I had no boundaries at all, be it with family or friends, I'd virtually allowed everyone around me to take advantage of the fact that I had none in place. I soon came to realise that I have nothing to feel guilty about and that by putting the strategies/tools into place that Kirsty gave me I have managed to rid myself of the events which occurred very early on in my life. I am now living my best life. When things start to feel a little tough, I now know what it is that I need to do. I now have a far better relationship with my whole family, son, mother and partner included. I have managed to disassociate myself from the negative people around me, I'm once again enjoying life very much! Thank you, Kirsty you are a truly inspirational woman.

1. CHAPTER ONE

1.1. INTRODUCTION

Hello, my name is Kirsty and for more than 15 years now, I have been fascinated by the mind and the hidden causes of pain – mentally, emotionally and physically. As is often the case, my discoveries came in the form of my own yearning to be free from suffering, which I now share with you in this book. If you would like to know more about my personal journey then I have shared more details at the end. However, I imagine, seeing as you are here and reading this, you are keen to know how to begin your own healing process. So, let's begin.

We all want to be happy and pain free but not many of us are living that experience. Why not? The natural tendency of the mind is to move towards greater happiness and the natural tendency of the body is to heal itself. Why is it then that don't we have constant happiness and health? In short, it is because we have forgotten our internal and natural mechanism for surrender and healing. We are always looking to the outside to fix our problems. We have developed a habit of resistance and getting in our own way and general confusion.

The intention of this book is to present a new way of thinking about your body and mind and the connection between the two. It is going to give you simple and practical tools to help you start taking control of your own physical, mental and emotional life. So simple, in fact, that it would be easy for you to dismiss the information here. I urge you, just for now, to set aside any judgements and read on with an open mind and an open heart.

Learning to meditate and then subsequently becoming a teacher of The Bright Path Ascension meditation practice has been one of the fundamental influences of my work. Clearly being able to see the correlation between our thinking patterns and behaviours and the effect they have on our health and wellbeing has given me the direct experience that if we want to be healthy, joyful and pain free, then we must work from the inside out. Not the other way around - as is prescribed by most modern medicine.

As a meditation teacher, one of the first questions we ask people is: "What is your highest desire on this planet?" Ultimately, whatever anyone says, it all leads back to the same answer. They may think they want a new car, a bigger house, better relationships, an exciting job etc. However, what underpins all these experiences is more peace, joy, and happiness.

This is possible. In fact, it is our birth right to live in freedom. We certainly have the choice of not settling for our present reality if it's painful. We can create a new one whenever we choose, but how many people truly and honestly believe that to be true? Interestingly, we are the only species on the planet that can think about a terrible outcome of a future event and by thought alone, we activate a chemical process in the body. We instantly release the stress hormone; cortisol. The most fascinating part about this is the subconscious mind thinks the event, conversation, experience we are thinking and focusing on is happening right now. The subconscious mind has no gauge on what's real and what's not. It can't differentiate between the two because it works more like a computer programme processing information.

It takes raw data from one end such as what you focus on, for example, thoughts, feelings, experiences, actions. It chews this up, filters it through all your other subconscious programmes and then acts. If the thoughts you are identified with are intensely negative, the subconscious mind will send signals to the rest of your body telling you that you are under attack or threat.

Amazing right? But what is infinitely more amazing is that we have the ability to unravel our destructive mental tendencies and create a life of joy and health by pure awareness or consciousness alone. Let me give you an example:

Recently, I had the pleasure of working with a retired Police Inspector who had been suffering from PTSD, chronic anxiety and depression for thirty years due to extreme trauma. He had been at the scene of a suicide thirty years prior where he had witnessed a father throw his three-year-old daughter from a 60 ft bridge and then jumped himself. Needless to say, the fatality was instant, however, the police Inspector had carried this horrific experience around with him, visiting the scene in his head every day since, blaming himself for what had happened, wishing he had done something different.

Over the years of him revisiting this story on a daily basis, not only was he literally re-living the experience from an internal world, but he was also cementing the memory in his subconscious. The rehearsal of this tragedy meant the body became the mind. As soon as his attention was put onto the story, the body instantly started to fire stress hormones. By the time I met him, he had tried working with a CBT practitioner, psychologist, counsellor and had untold appointments with doctors for medication; none of which had managed to stop his PTSD, anxiety and depression. The problem is that the focus had been on anxiety and depression (the symptoms), rather than identifying the cause and letting that go.

Regrettably, many healing modalities focus on trying to fix a person who isn't actually broken. There may be a perception that they are broken. But this couldn't be further from the truth. No one is broken, you may believe you are but you are NOT! This is very significant, as most people I meet think there is something wrong with them. Their back, their body, their mind, their life etc. When in fact, like a stuck record all that's happened is they are replaying negative programming and negative stories in their mind, which triggers negative emotion. This then manifests in the body and creates a reality which makes a person seem broken.

In the case of the wonderful Police Inspector he had a belief that he was broken when I met him too. He was also very well-rehearsed as he had been replaying the story of that tragic event and associated feelings, every day for thirty years. It had almost become his identity, to the point that his mind started to fix the event onto comparisons in his own family, Such as aligning the little girl who tragically died with his own daughter, who was also three, at the time. This gave him the chance to punish himself even more. Every milestone, every event, would be another chance to go over it in his mind. It became like an addiction. As long as he was torturing himself by reliving the event in his mind, he unconsciously felt like he was at least taking some responsibility for the pain himself. This distracted him away from the feelings of guilt for a moment, even though he had absolutely nothing to be guilty for. Of course, he did everything and more to try and save the little girl.

Once he saw the truth that it was out of his control and he wasn't to blame, he could then through the Freedom Alignment Method, allow himself to let go of all the suppressed/repressed emotions around this traumatic event and rewrite his story.

Today, he is like a new man at 70! In his words, he said: "I'm finally free of feeling trapped by anxiety and stress and I can, for the first time in 30 years, speak about it without breaking down."

The question is:

» Why do we hold onto trauma, stress, pain and bad experiences?
» Is it a conscious choice?
» This is a big question which I will answer throughout the book.

But ask yourself this:

» Why would I hold onto things that are negative and sad?
» Why would I revisit it in my mind over and over again if it only ever makes me feel terrible?

Please keep reading if you want to know the answer.

1.2. WHO IS THIS BOOK FOR?

Are you suffering from chronic physical or emotional pain? Are you so anxious that you can't seem to live your life without a feeling of crippling dread? Do you have paralysing emotional pain, a prolonged illness or are experiencing a long recovery from an injury? Are you in chronic pain or suffering from stress and anxiety? Are you someone that hasn't had a decent night's sleep in years? Are you someone who has become a slave to pharmaceutical drugs, alcohol, street drugs, excessive shopping, excessive spending or has an unhealthy relationship with food?

If you can answer yes to any of these questions then this book is for you. If you have answered no then perhaps you know someone who has experienced these feelings?

The book has been written to show you that there is an underlying cause to your physical, mental and emotional pain that you might not be aware of. It will support you to start today to realign with your natural state of homeostasis, presence and health.

And, by the way, I am not here to tell you that your pain and illness is all in your head. No, it is very real. And I'm definitely not here to say that other modalities like Western medication don't have a place. In acute situations, I think that pharmaceutical drugs are an absolute must.

However, I would ask; are they addressing the root cause or is it merely an Elastoplast? I totally understand why someone would take medication when there is so much pain to deal with and they don't know that there is another way. I am not a medical doctor so I would always strongly recommend that you seek advice from your doctor once you have read this book and before implementing the tools. Once you have done this, you are then ready to start reducing your load.

1.3. HOW TO USE THIS BOOK

The first step of this journey is to give you some necessary knowledge. This may not be your normal reading or information but bear with me, it's necessary so that you can take the steps to make the relevant changes to create the life you deserve. There are some fundamental shifts that will start to happen as you go through the pages.

I want you to become aware of your thoughts and emotions while reading this book. You will see that every exercise I ask you to complete is NOT difficult but it IS different. There may be a conflict or a pull to judge the information before putting it into action. It may be that you feel excited or angry when reading some of the information contained herein. That's ok, just remember to keep an open heart and an open mind.

In order to get results, you MUST complete all of the questions and exercises. Consistency is key; I cannot emphasise that enough. Just like going to the gym, if you go once you will feel great after that session but won't reap the long-term benefits. However, if you go to the gym consistently you will be fitter, healthier and feel good. This process is no different. If you do the exercises once, you will get some awareness and shift but not necessarily the results you're looking for. If you are willing to make it a priority and be consistent with the exercises you will reap huge rewards.

The more severe your pain, the more letting go there is to do. Don't listen to your mind if it says "this is not working." This is your egoic mind going into panic as you start to break through old behaviours, repressed emotions and beliefs. The key thing to remember is that as adults we learn through repetition. Through repeating the exercises over and over you will gain the results you are looking for. Resist the temptation to skip ahead. There may be a desire to jump to a part of the book that you think sounds interesting or is addressing something you have not heard of before. You might just want to cut to the chase and get on with the exercises. I get it, I have that kind of mind too. It is critical and judgemental and often talks to me, like it knows it all. I ask that you're extremely vigilant in this process. Read each section, even if you already know about that subject. A wise man once told me, "you don't know what you don't know." Therefore, you may never know what you may need reminding of. Or even more importantly, there may be a new perspective, tool or action which will help you overcome your pain once and for all.

Throughout this book I will be asking you to write down your thoughts or feelings on several subjects. I suggest you get a notebook to write these things in so that you can keep them all together and reflect upon them later. The reason for writing your thoughts down is to begin to access a deeper truth held within the subconscious mind. Writing is the fastest way to tap into this and the fastest way to tap into your subconscious mind, is through writing. It distracts you from working things out from your intellect. Sometimes it can take a few minutes of writing before the truth starts to flow, be patient. We call this a stream of consciousness. A great tip to consider when asking yourself a question such as: "why am I feeling angry," is to write down whatever comes to mind. Keep writing until you have nothing left to write. Do not overthink the process just allow the pen to flow. It may or may not even make sense. This does not matter, as this is all about transference of energy. The best thing you can do is not read through it as you are writing, save that until you have finished the exercise. Again, when you do read back through it, please do not overthink everything you have written. Trust that whatever has appeared is correct. The fundamental part of this exercise is that you are not doing it from your mind. You are accessing a flow from your sub conscious mind.

Lastly, I don't profess to know it all. However, after studying the relationship between the body, mind and emotions for more than 15 years – personally through my own inner experience, academically and practically through the observation of thousands of clients – I know that the Freedom Alignment Method, which I present to you within this book, works, so please give it a try.

One last point before we dive in. You must forgive me for this. You will find that I repeat certain key points throughout the pages - it is intentional! Repetition is key to creating new neural pathways of understanding. If new information is not revisited within 80 minutes of learning it will fade away and leave your short-term memory. We forget most information we are exposed to because the brain has been developed to do this so that important current information can have access with ease. Generally, the day to day information we are exposed to is unimportant, however if you do desire to move information from short term memory into long term memory then we need to repeat and connect the information to previous knowledge. Therefore, stopping every now and then to revisit the information in your mind is a very good thing. Every time we learn something new our brain forms new connections, neurons and makes existing neural pathways stronger or weaker. What fires together wires together!

2. CHAPTER TWO UNDERSTANDING PAIN

2.1. WHAT IS PAIN?

There are two ways to look at pain. Firstly, you touch a hot oven. Immediately a signal travels quickly through nerve fibres up into the brain which triggers a reaction for you to pull your hand away, to avoid burning yourself. Secondly, you're about to go to a job interview, your stomach is churning and you feel nauseous. These physical feelings of pain or discomfort are triggered through thought. Here is the kicker, there is actually a third cause of physical chronic pain.

This is the sole driving force for encouraging me to put pen to paper around this topic.

From an anatomical point of view, physical pain happens when a change in the body's nervous system occurs. To be more accurate, it is a constriction of the blood vessels that reduces blood flow to the muscles and nerves of the body, caused when we have a reaction to stimulus which we label as negative and unwanted. This leads to us resisting the negative feeling which literally cuts off oxygen to these areas and causes a blockage. This is what causes the physical sensation of pain.

Mostly we spend our lives trying to escape any type of pain. We go to school and then start working super hard so we can guarantee we won't feel the pain of being unemployed and broke when we can't get a well-paid job. We try to be as careful as possible selecting a husband or wife/partner so we don't have to feel the pain of loneliness, rejection and the potential of experiencing a broken heart. We get married in order to guarantee we won't feel the pain of separation. We take medication, pain killers or street drugs so we don't have to feel emotional and or physical pain in our mind and or our body. We save money like crazy for our future so we don't have to feel the pain of working forever. We limit our intake of fun. We end up taking life so seriously that it becomes our default setting because we have bought into the illusion that this makes us a responsible model citizen. In this situation the pain comes from fear, fear of judgment by our society, our peers.

If you take a close look at your life you will see it is designed specifically to avoid pain. If you have ever experienced anything traumatic; a loss of a pet, a relationship break-up, financial issues, arguments, a wedding (stress and trauma doesn't always come from a negative experience), job change, house move, a death in the family, a friendship break-up and the list goes on. Chances are you never really fully processed all of the uncomfortable feelings that these events provoked. It is likely that you repressed or suppressed the emotion which accompanied the event, person or place. This is not your fault. You are hardwired, just like every organism on this planet, for the continual reassuring movement away from pain and towards pleasure.

This is why the heroin addict will behave in a way which seems inhumane, such as to steal from an old lady, family member or friend, not because they are innately bad, but because the pain of needing that next fix is so great, they are prepared to do whatever it takes. Even if the behaviour they undertake was once something they would have never dreamt of doing. In fact, pain itself is not the problem, it's actually the meaning that we attach to it that causes resistance and subsequently feeds the pain.

Once meaning is added to the pain, we then experience resistance. It is important to remember here, "that which we resist, persists." Most of us are absolutely terrified of pain because of what we have determined pain to mean. Generally speaking, we all have beliefs about pain that we downloaded from our parents when we were very young.

I want you to ask yourself the following question and answer as honestly as possible, writing the answer in your notebook:

2.2. WHAT DOES PAIN MEAN?

Ask yourself the question and then see what comes out of your pen without thinking about it. As I said, like a stream of consciousness. Allow the real truth of your meaning towards this word to flow through your pen. The actual truth of what pain means to you is not anything you should judge as good or bad. For many of you it will be the first time you have ever asked yourself what meaning have I given to this word, "pain." So please do not take this as an opportunity to be hard on yourself. The key importance of this exercise is what you do with the answer.

Now you have your meaning of pain. Here are some examples of the meaning we give to pain.

"I don't like it; this needs to stop"

"Why me, it is not fair"

"I hate hurting"

"It is a bad thing"

"I am broken"

"My body lets me down"

"I am scared that I will always be like this"

"It's so hard"

"I can't stand living like this"

Then ask the question, is the meaning you have given to pain, in other words, are your beliefs about pain, serving you? When I refer to the word "serving" in this context it means something which is supportive and positive to your greater need. For example, something that creates a positive feeling inside like eating healthy, moving your body and being grateful for life. I also use the word "resisting or resistance" which means in this case something you are pushing against like an experience or emotion which you deem uncomfortable or bad. In other words, does the meaning (belief) lead you to greater freedom, joy etc. or the opposite?

Is the definition you have given to pain serving you? Let's assume you have made the meaning of pain the enemy. In other words, it is not serving you. At this point you may be feeling slightly confused - why wouldn't you think pain is bad when it hurts so much! One very significant reason would be that pain is the mechanism that allows you to know that you have something you need to see, let go of or allow. In this sense it is ACTUALLY a gift, this is a key learning.

Please answer the following questions, do not overthink the answer, write down the first thing that comes to mind even if it does not make sense to you. Grab your book and pen and answer with openness and innocence.

- Is the meaning you have given to pain outdated? In other words, after reading a short way into this book are you starting to change your opinion about pain?
- If so, does it need updating?

- If it does need updating then do it. Rewrite the meaning you have attributed to pain. Do this by writing a statement in the present tense (because your subconscious mind has no idea what is real and what isn't) that serves your greater good. Refer to my point above, could pain be a gift?
- In my experience, there was a time I had an epiphany whereby I realised that a previous abusive relationship was the catalyst for how I behave now. This pain was my gift. Let me explain. What I experienced in the relationship was a catalyst for my own transformation and so became the gift. This became apparent to me as a new opportunity to learn to become more aware of my actions in life, experiencing more of life from the present moment and learning how to shift my vibration into one of unconditional love. This meant only one thing; that I became more aware of what was really going on. This became intoxicating as I realised that this was not only the case for myself but for all my clients too. It was at this point I coined the phrase "pain is the gift."

2.3. PHYSICAL PAIN

Physical pain is what most of us understand pain to be. We fall over, it hurts. We cut ourselves, it hurts. We break a bone, it hurts. Physical pain is simply a physical cause and effect. However, alongside physical pain, we also experience emotional and or mental pain – which of course, can also be "felt" as a physical experience within the body. However, the trigger for most chronic physical pain (with some small exceptions) is due to strong suppressed negative emotions that cause an inflammatory response in the body.

2.4. EMOTIONAL PAIN

Emotional pain happens when we identify with low vibrational emotions such as shame, guilt, fear, apathy, jealousy or anger. It is the illusion that we are out of control. What I mean by "out of control," is that we tend to have a negative belief, opinion or perspective of a meaning we give something in our objective world only when the emotions are low vibrational. This consequently gives you an experience that feels heavy and downward spiralling in that moment. Emotional pain does not have a physical or external cause but rather a feeling of uncomfortableness that arises because of an attachment to a negative thought process. Therefore, emotional pain arrives when we are out of alignment with our truth; out of alignment with our higher self.

Continual experience of emotional pain is due to the suppressed emotions within the subconscious mind. These suppressed emotions will surface on a reoccurring basis until you let them go. However, most people don't realise this because the mechanism of a human is to move from pain to pleasure unconsciously and at all costs. The person will naturally stuff the negative emotion back down, usually through avoidance behaviours such as overspending, overeating, drinking, sex, gossiping, gambling, T.V. etc.

These behaviours are created to allow us to move out of the feeling of pain. We do this automatically without any realisation we are doing it - until we become aware of this. Up until that point you will find that you will keep manifesting situations and scenarios in your life that reflect these negative suppressed emotions. An example could be someone who is suppressing negative emotions such as fear, guilt and anger. They have multiple romantic relationships where they create or manifest the same problems but with different people. This will continue to happen until the focus is taken away from the external relationship and put on the internal relationship and the negative repressed or suppressed emotion. Only then will they stop recreating the same patterns of behaviour.

2.5. MENTAL PAIN

Mental psychological pain is intense and can seem insufferable at times. Mental pain is emotionally based and has the ability to trigger thoughts and feelings of suffering which exist in the mind and body. Most people's relationship to mental pain is a reflection of their programmes, belief systems, values, experiences and memories held in the unconscious mind. Mental pain is triggered unconsciously by the five senses - seeing somebody you haven't seen for a while, smelling something, hearing something, touching something and or having a flashback memory etc. Mental pain feels significant as, just like physical and emotional pain, it is uncomfortable and can have a huge impact on the ways you interact with the world. I often see a common theme with clients experiencing mental pain in that there has been a time lapse where the person hasn't updated their meanings as to how something feels. An example of this is when you find yourself reacting to someone at work. Perhaps the reaction was over the top, you finally take a breath and calm down. At that point, if you were to ask yourself "does the behaviour warrant the reaction?" you would find in some cases, that it is old programming, perhaps it had triggered an old feeling or experience which then re-ignited all the fire and wrath of the past. This was then projected onto the person at work, and it wasn't really much to do with the current situation at all.

2.6. THE RELATIONSHIP BETWEEN PHYSICAL, EMOTIONAL AND MENTAL PAIN - HOW WE AVOID IT!

We all have a natural tendency to move away from pain. It is a human survival mechanism. Sigmund Freud contrived the "The pain pleasure principle."

He said that this suggested that people are always making choices to ensure they avoid pain or make choices that increase pleasure. It should be noted that "The pain pleasure principle" is the influence of all the decisions we make. We are a collection of principles that are influenced by our beliefs, perspectives, values and decisions. This has a direct reflection on the way we interpret pain and pleasure. Mainly based on our past experience and upbringing. Whether we are aware of it or not, we seek pleasure for the reward of instant gratification. However, Freud also highlighted that we seek to AVOID PAIN. Interestingly, while working with clients, I see them continually swerve any form of conflict because they hate confrontation. What is fascinating to highlight is that they have associated confrontation with a feeling of discomfort (pain)? And so, will do anything to avoid it, sometimes at the cost of their own sanity and health. Even if the situation is unhealthy and negative, they would rather stay in that situation than face the fear of dealing with it.

2.7. WHAT DOES PAIN MEAN TO ME?

To me, personally, pain meant rejection. A common relationship to pain is the belief that if you do something wrong or get something wrong then it must be changed. If not, pain will lead you to believe that you were unlovable, unaccepted or even worse not wanted. The subsequent feeling is that of rejection.

Humans are a social species. We unconsciously mirror each other's emotions, neurones, movement and brain activity, all of the time. The thought of rejection to the egoic mind is equal to that of death. In fact, being isolated from others for most people is worse than death. So, if the meaning of pain is rejection then we become terrified of the path that leads to the feeling of rejection.

We haven't just done this with pain. We have also created programmes around other negative emotions such as anger. It's so common that many of us as small children were told not to be angry as it is unacceptable or told that BEING angry is unacceptable. We learnt very quickly to stop expressing these emotions, as it could result in rejection or lack of love and connection from our parents or guardians.

If you received that message as a child, then unconsciously, you have made feeling pain wrong and therefore bad, the moment you feel pain, guess what? You will try and push it away. You will resist it by trying desperately to control external conditions so you never feel pain again. In fact, all this does is cause more pain. Any trauma or emotion that comes up that we do not or have not processed will leave an imprint in the mind and body. This always has a story, narrative or dialogue, be it out loud or in the head. Most humans unconsciously tell their story daily as it becomes their focal point and identity. It is often based on being a victim and this fuels the pain.

2.8. WHAT IS THE PURPOSE OF PAIN?

As I mentioned at the beginning of this chapter, pain is a multidimensional experience on a physical, emotional and mental level. Regardless of where you see this pain starting it will involve all three aspects at times. Its purpose is to get your attention. I heard someone say the other day "suffering is grace unfolding." I love this, as I've always seen pain as the roadmap to the experience of more joy. In other words, pain is the doorway to enlightenment. To make it go away should not be our goal. We need to let the pain reveal to us what needs to be "shown and known." So that we can return to homeostasis or health.

Pain is the first crucial component of healing. It allows us to search for the cause. The underpinning of what's really going on. When we identify the cause, we have to face the fears that are inherent within our body and our being. We have to face what we have almost certainly been trying to avoid, albeit unconsciously. We have to feel it and deal with it as opposed to trying to avoid it.

In my experience, the suppressed emotions of anger and rage are one of the primary causes of pain and must be faced. I will explain this in more detail later on. Often, these emotions can be so well hidden that the person who inhabits this type of emotion in their subconscious mind can sometimes appear pretty relaxed. Therefore, they might find it hard to believe that they have spent a lifetime stuffing these types of emotions away. They have no idea that they are angry. But let's face it, if, as a child, you learned that being angry was wrong, you'd learn pretty fast to stuff that away if it meant being accepted and loved.

Interestingly, pain will intensify the more you resist, perhaps you've been asked to do something you do NOT want to do. You may decide to do it anyway but as a result you will feel resistance or frustration. Your body will react to this in some way. It might be something obvious such as tense shoulders or clenched teeth, it might be something less so, such as a headache or feeling nauseous. Next time you are faced with this dilemma, be aware of what you're being asked to do, to say or to help with. Notice what it is that you're feeling and therefore resisting, especially when the pain increases. You'll notice that your mind will immediately shift your attention onto your body when you have a strong desire to NOT do that thing. Where are you feeling it in your body? This is a huge sign that inwards there is something you are now ready to see and let go of. Your body is telling you that you are not living your truth. For example: You know there is a difficult conversation to be had. You find yourself starting with a migraine or intense headache before even being in the same room as the person. This is due to the resistance it creates which then manifests in the body.

Trying to avoid the signals pain is giving you can take over your life. Pain gets your attention. The body talks, but mostly we ignore it and then try and push it away. In reality, all we need to ask is "what do I need to see, let go of or be ok with?" Then see what arises. Only then is it time to rest into what lies underneath the pain. I will help you learn how to do this in subsequent chapters.

The first step is to know that there is a negative emotion directly underneath the pain even if you think that your shoulder is hurting because of your posture or some other reason. If the pain changes in severity and or changes location in the body for example, firstly there is pain in your shoulder, next it's in your upper back, then it moves back into the shoulder and so on and so forth is a sure sign that the physical pain has been emotionally triggered. We need to find the negative emotion beneath the pain. This is the fastest way to change your relationship to it. Only then can healing take place and pain subside. However, even this can be a trap. You have to be ok if it stays or if it goes. No attachment to anything. Only then do you stop trying to control your circumstances which will result in all suffering eventually evaporating. Sometimes we may distract ourselves from the pain momentarily but unless the core issue is headed on, the pain will return. It returns to tell you there is more "processing" still to be done.

2.9. SECONDARY GAINS TO PAIN: WHAT IS A SECONDARY GAIN?

Secondary gains occur when there is a conscious or unconscious driver that outweighs the benefit of being in pain. This can be a hard pill to swallow, can be classed as chronic pain and is so exhausting, debilitating and miserable. Why would you wish it upon yourself? Ok, let us start with a fact, you are NOT a failure. You have done this unconsciously. You have only done it because there is a person, situation, belief or need that isn't being met and the desire for this is so great that you manifest a secondary gain.

Some common secondary gains could be:

- Feeling better after taking medication - a relief to being dependant on prescription drugs with the excuse to use them.
- A sense of approval or validation from the doctor who has given you a label to justify your state.
- An escape from having to face more responsibilities.
- Much needed rest, you feel exhausted and don't feel like you can stop unless you are ill.
- An excuse to escape sexual demands from a partner.
- Physical pain acting as a relief or distraction from overwhelming emotional pain.
- Much desired attention from others, like your partner, work colleagues, family.
- Money, you get to have more benefits for being ill.
- An excuse to avoid working in an unsatisfying, depressing job.
- A stressful employment situation you don't want to face.
- Your identity of being the sick member of the family. Who will you be if you're not that label? The illness gives you some purpose at least!

I do not want you to beat yourself up if there is a secondary gain. This is only about gaining awareness to what is really going on. At the same time there may be a natural defence mechanism to want to dismiss this section. If that is what you are feeling right now then STOP. You are about to have a breakthrough. The journey of truth can sometimes feel uncomfortable. That's ok, just rest into this experience without judgment. At the other side of this is freedom. It is now time for you to do some writing in your notebook. Ask yourself:

What benefits am I getting from being stuck with my pain? Be it an illness, emotional, mental, physical or disease? What are the benefits of being out of ease with oneself?

Be as honest as you can be, as it will serve you in the long run. It does not make you a manipulative person if you have been buying into any of the above drivers for secondary gains. It makes you very human. Secondary gains are self-sabotaging and often the biggest hurdle for healing. The key here is the initial awareness. Nine times out of ten they are unconscious motivators which allow the person to feel a reward in one way or another. They show you that the pain is there to help you meet a basic human need.

I have often seen this with clients who come to me with illnesses such as Fibromyalgia. In many cases, there is a conscious or unconscious desire to be loved. This can often look like the person feels sorry for themselves, which can be quite rightly justified as Fibromyalgia is so painful. In order to move through this illness, this "victim mentality" has to be shifted. This opens the person up to the potential that they have been holding onto a belief that the attention they are receiving because of the pain is better than no attention. Of course, the severity of impact based on this belief varies vastly between clients.

Those who see it, are prepared to change their behaviours, let go of their guilt and trust that they are loved, get better. But not everyone is ready to do this. The ego would have you believe that you would do anything to be out of pain. So why would you create your own suffering in order to get love? You often find that people's reasons are so obscured from their view due to their coping mechanisms, that they also grab onto the illness and the labels that accompany them. This gives the person something worth living for, a life purpose, even if it is negative.

A common negative suppressed emotion that often triggers a secondary gain is anger. The reason people hold onto anger is that it gives them a sense of power, which often covers up their inability to have clear and appropriate boundaries. The anger makes the person feel safe. The actual behaviour that needs working on is boundary setting. Once this is addressed and the negative emotion is let go of then the pain will disappear. Think back to the question I set above regarding doing something you do not want to do. I can almost guarantee that you felt anger. Doing something you really don't want to, pushes against your boundaries. You feel powerless in it; anger helps redress that balance because you don't realise there is another way.

One of the biggest challenges I see with secondary gains is that the hidden benefits are so self-serving to that person, they don't want to acknowledge that this is even possible. Not taking responsibility allows the person to keep on blaming and stops them having to look at their circumstances and behaviours. The truth is when we take responsibility it empowers us and this is often an integral part of the healing process.

2.10. THE DIFFERENCE BETWEEN PAIN AND SUFFERING

Pain happens in the moment; suffering is the story we wrap around the pain which intensifies it and keeps it in play. Attachment is a good example of suffering. Attachment is when the mind makes something personal. The ups and downs of life are inevitable, but when we are attached to a certain outcome and it doesn't go our way, our mind will tell us that we will never get over this, it isn't fair, why me? etc. This is the narrative which causes us to suffer.

Pain is the body's signal that there is something out of alignment with your truth. Or in other words, you are out of homeostasis. When someone is experiencing pain and is resistant to it, this will result in suffering, every single time. The longer the person resists the experience the more intense the pain and more prolonged the suffering. The resistance itself will cause more of the stress hormone, cortisol, in the body. This is like pouring fuel over a fire when someone is in pain.

Mostly, humans suffer because they are unconscious to their attachment to the story they have wrapped around the pain. Pain is definitely real but there is a tendency to go into fixing it rather than being ok with it and actually FEELING the underlying emotion which is fuelling the pain. When we feel, we go from resisting it to allowing it. Only then can healing take place. You will never heal so long as you are in survival mode.

It's pretty fair to say that all humans will experience some pain in their lives. Suffering is an option though. Pain can show up through losing a loved one, an accident, a past trauma which has never been processed. This may sit dormant in the subconscious mind as suppressed emotions. I remember my first ever boyfriend moving to London to go to university. At the time the 250 miles distance was too big for us to continue, so we parted. My heart literally ached with pain. I honestly don't think I was ever the same again after this experience. But because I was so young my life and attention moved on to the next moment with general ease. So suffering wasn't my experience at all. I felt sad and cried for the first 24 hours solidly. Then life presented new opportunities, friends and a new direction. As much as he had a special place in my heart and still does today, I didn't keep going back to "but what if", I moved forward with excitement.

It is possible to be in pain and not suffer and it is also possible to suffer without physical pain. Make change your friend. Suffering is the resistance of that which is painful. When you let go of the resistance to pain it loses the capacity to make you suffer. Suffering is not natural, it's always out of choice that we suffer.

Pain is a natural process of the body - it's very good for you. It tells you that there is some danger, threat and letting go to do. The benefits of pain are that it stops you from doing things that aren't good for you. It allows you to know what is right and wrong. It's a great communication tool. Suffering is a psychological thing. You can either suffer or not it's YOUR choice. You may want to reread this paragraph again; suffering is a CHOICE!

Learning how to change your relationship to emotions and thoughts is paramount to peace. If you can create suffering you can also create the opposite.

2.11. WHY DOES IT FEEL SO HARD TO CHANGE?

It seems like it is so hard to change as most people unconsciously revert back into habitual daily thoughts, emotions and behaviours. The only way to create change is to do something different. Which makes sense when you think about it because what you have been trying, clearly hasn't been working. Yet we keep on doing the same things. Partly because we haven't seen this until now. We believe that it is the only option, however, a belief is merely a thought we have thought several times.

The great news is it's impossible to go backwards. There may be a perception that you've gone back but this isn't actually true. Once you are consciously aware of the things you do, and the world around you; there is no backwards. There is only ever forwards from that moment on.

2.12. WHAT IS STRESS AND WHY DO WE NEED IT?

"Stress is determined by our belief systems and their associated emotional pressures. It is not the external stimulus, then, that is the cause of stress, but our degree of reactivity. The more surrendered we are, the

less prone we are to stress. The damage caused by stress is merely the result of our own emotions."

Dr David Hawkins - Letting Go - The Pathway to Surrender

Stress is neither good nor bad; it is the response to tell you that you're out of balance; out of homeostasis.

"Homeostasis is the ability to maintain a relatively stable internal state that persists despite changes in the world outside. All living organisms, from plants to puppies to people, must regulate their internal environment to process energy and ultimately survive."

By livescience

2.13. THE SCIENCE BEHIND THE THEORY

The body's sympathetic nervous system will always activate in response to acute stress. This happens due to a sudden release of hormones, such as cortisol and adrenaline. It starts with the fact that your body is reacting continuously to your thoughts and feelings, which in turn fires chemicals off throughout the mind and body. Since the mind and body are connected, you never experience one without the other. These transmitters are called neuropeptides (a chemical signal in the form of protein like molecules used by neurones to communicate with each other). This is the communication tool between all the cells of the body.

On average the human body has around 50 trillion cells which are fully replaced every two months and they operate as a community. Each cell works independently and together. They have their own reproductive system, nervous system and digestive system. The neuropeptides communicate through receptor cells into the cell itself and this influences the behaviour of the cell. Our cells are like mini humans without heads. They simulate all the systems we have as a human. I am also intrigued by the way they communicate, reproduce and efficiently work as different departments in a team format to keep you alive. All of which is done without you having to consciously think about it. Some examples of neuropeptides are Endorphins (adrenaline), GABA, Acetylcholine, Dopamine and Serotonin.

Since the mind and body are completely connected, when neuropeptides are released you experience it in both the brain and the physical body. The neuropeptides have different qualities depending on the thoughts and feelings you're focusing on. All cells are covered in receptors which translate the information. Very quickly they pass on the message that you're happy or sad.

The limbic system (which is also called the emotional centre of the brain) is where the hypothalamus, a gland which translates emotions into physical responses, lives. It also has other jobs, like overseeing your blood sugar levels, body temperature, controlling your appetite, looking after your heart and lungs, your digestive system etc. The limbic system is like a pharmacy, releasing neuropeptides when necessary and lives in the Amygdala which is recognised for being connected to fear and or any pleasure you experience.

It's also where the pineal gland lives. The pineal gland has a very important role, it monitors the hormone system and releases natural pain killers/ antidepressants when necessary such as endorphins. All of this lives in the frontal portion of the temporal lobe. The sympathetic nervous system starts to stimulate the adrenal glands which result in an increase of blood pressure, breathing and heart rate.

This is when you physically start to think there is something seriously wrong. Especially if you don't know that it's a chemical response to your thoughts. 16 years ago, I suffered with intense anxiety and panic attacks. At the time I had no understanding of how to deal with the way I was feeling. They would impact my life to the point I would think that I was dying. I have clients, who in the past, found themselves in A&E because their hearts were pounding so fast, they thought they were having a heart attack. The thoughts that accompany these types of experiences are usually ones of pure terror.

It takes a human about 20 to 60 minutes after the acute stress response is activated, to settle. The stressful thoughts and chemicals such as cortisol continue after the event is over. If you engage in the thought then the body will keep reacting to the thought like the event is still actually happening, even if it's just in your mind. The reason for this, as mentioned before is because the subconscious mind has no ability to discern what is happening in real life, real time to what is happening in your imagination.

Also, as mentioned before, unlike other organisms on the planet, we are the only ones able to trigger the stress hormone from thought alone. We are also unlike any other organism, who, after a stressful physical or mental experience, don't shake the cortisol out of the body. A zebra for example, who is being chased by a tiger and in this case is lucky to get away, will spend a few minutes shaking after the experience to release the stress hormone out of their body. Once it has done this it will then return back to grazing as though nothing has happened.

The frontal lobe of a human is 40% larger than any other mammal. This allows us to look back on our life events, which can cause us to feel depressed. Depression is triggered when someone is lost in thought and emotion from the past. Anxiety is when someone is a future worrier and gets lost in future negative fantasy, often based on bad past experiences or frightening TV, news stories etc. which they catapult into a future moment and attach to their life, even though it is not their reality.

These two behaviours are usually unconscious and very addictive. I've never worked with or met anyone to date who is suffering from acute anxiety and or depression who is anchored or resting in the present moment. They are always lost in a story of "what if's" or drawn to their body functions, a racing heartbeat, an increase in the body's temperature and or muscle tension. Humans will revisit the event/story in their heads time and time again. Sometimes for days, weeks, years or even a lifetime. People will hold grudges, not let things go and become obsessed with being right.

The problem is, every time you engage in the story and or memory in your mind, and because the subconscious mind has no idea what's real and what's not, it goes into survival mode. Immediately, the mind signals to the body that there is a threat and like the obedient servant, it sends a signal to the mind body and now the chemistry of the body and the thoughts of the mind are off again.

The stress response is automatically released so the body starts to experience a flood of cortisol ready to fight for its survival. Truthfully though you've been sitting in your front room on your sofa, watching an episode of "Game of Thrones" while your mind has drifted off into an argument you had three days ago with someone and now, you're going over how angry you are at this person who said something you didn't like. You even start imagining a fake scenario in your head, going back over what you would really have loved to have said to this person. All the while, your subconscious mind thinks this argument in your mind is actually happening now. We sometimes call the acute stress trigger "fight or flight." This occurs in times which are deemed as threatening or terrifying even if they are only in our imagination!

It is worth noting that human beings still operate a stone age hunter gatherer mindset. We are hardwired to a brain which still operates in the same way as it did when humans first walked this planet. In simple terms it means that because our world has changed dramatically, we no longer need a "fight or flight" response to go hunting for our food; we have supermarkets! However, the mind does not know this and so the "fight or flight" response is triggered, perhaps because you are focused on overwhelm or you feel like you have too much to do, maybe you have just had an intense argument or maybe you are experiencing some general day to day stress. The crazy part of the mind - body response is no different to being a caveman who once did have to run for his life due to some wild animal chasing him for their dinner.

2.14. WHAT ARE FEELINGS AND SENSATIONS?

A feeling is a subjective conscious experience. Sensations are external, such as pulsing, heat, tingling, pressure etc. It is the brain's way of giving meaning based on past experiences. This is attached to the feeling or emotion.

2.15. WHAT IS AN EMOTION?

Emotions vary from downward spiralling/negative ones such as anger, fear, sadness etc to upward spiralling and positive ones such as love and joy. The difference between emotions and feelings is that emotions manifest subconsciously. They are spontaneous physiological reactions to objective experiences that we have in our day to day lives. They are literally "energy in motion," "E Motion." We experience feelings consciously and have thousands of feelings, yet only a handful of emotions. Many people experience their entire life never understanding their feelings and emotions. Interestingly I recognise in clients regularly, the belief that negative emotions and feelings are bad, when in fact they are just a communication tool to tell the person that they are out of alignment with homeostasis. Something in their life needs to be addressed. Perhaps they have been putting up with something in their objective world that is not what they want. It could be a destructive relationship or even the habit of not being able to say "no" because of a feeling of guilt and or fear. Unfortunately, the side effect of this is that resentment bubbles away in the subconscious mind. Often the person is not aware of this until it's too late, they then begin to manifest anxiety, depression or potentially chronic pain. Or perhaps they find themselves in a situation with a person where they are not saying what they really feel. All these different types of experiences trigger suppressed negative emotions and feelings. You must be able to remember a time when someone has said something to you in a situation where you have strongly felt it was better to not say how you truly felt as it wasn't worth the argument. The emotion then gets ignored which is fine if it's the only time this has ever happened. However human behaviour shows us that how you do one thing is how you do everything. Therefore, the person who says "yes" when they really mean "no" or the person who keeps quiet instead of saying what they really feel, begins to create suppressed negative emotions which live in the subconscious mind. Again, this generally only gets the person's attention once they start to manifest anxiety, physical pain, illness. The choice is then taken out of the person's hands.

An example of this is: DISAPPOINTMENT, FEAR & GUILT vs OPTIMISM

» Disappointment, fear and guilt are NOT emotions you want to get good at. However, many of us have become experts at them.
» Telling people YOUR disappointing, negative stories on repeat are NOT the ones you want to focus on. If you notice you are doing this then STOP and bear in mind, "where attention goes energy flows."
» Disappointment takes you into the past, it pulls you into a story which can only ever result in you giving your power way. Fear, keeps you trapped in an illusion of your own mind. "False Evidence Appearing Real." Guilt not only keeps you unconscious, it will eat you alive, make you ill and create resentment.
» However, optimism takes you into the NOW where all YOUR power and human potential lives.

The thrill of life is being on the brink of that next explosion into another expansive experience, the next realisation of a big knowing, a large understanding, a huge intuitive download - don't you love being alive? Then focus on the MOTION of an upward spiralling vibration. This creates a positive "E motion." Which is energy in motion. Become aware of what comes out of your mouth! It's key to your next- level shift. Many people are not listening to the language they use about themselves. Become aware of this and you will be shocked at the amount of "I need to," "I can't," "I don't have enough." All hidden contracts to the universe that you're not enough, not worthy enough, do not deserve it or do not believe it is possible. So, begin with getting more aware of where you are putting your attention. It is key to change.

This is the difference between ease/flow and hardship/pain.

2.16. WHAT IS A THOUGHT?

A thought is a mental process that allows humans to create a reality and navigate as effectively and efficiently as possible as they can according to their desires. A thought is not the mind, it is a product of the mind.

2.17. WHAT IS THINKING?

When someone is in a thinking process, they are manipulating information through concepts, problem solving and decision making, based on programmes, memories and data that they have unconsciously downloaded, generally before the age of seven. Thinking is a stream of thought. It takes you out of being here, now in the present state and takes you into a past or a future moment. Thought is harmless and is a by-product of the brain in action. When we are unconsciously in a thinking process it causes stress on the nervous system because our mind and body are connected.

2.18. THOUGHTS AND FEELINGS

Thoughts and feelings keep us trapped in the same behaviours and actions which in turn creates the same reality. Mostly, people are unconscious to their thoughts which are largely influenced by their habits, beliefs and programmes, all of which live in the subconscious mind. It can seem like we are our thoughts and feelings but this is not true. Since we can observe our thoughts and feelings, we cannot be them. That would be like saying I can observe my car, dog and house and I am them. You know if you can observe something it is objective to you. This is great news since the average person has over 70,000 thoughts per day. Which I know sounds like a lot, it is! However, thoughts are not the enemy until we grab them and make them personal to us. Then they seemingly feel very real and very quickly they begin to consume us. This is generally because the thought or the thinking story which you go off into is familiar. You have thought about it many times before. Humans are habitual creatures and 90% of what you think about today you will think about tomorrow.

A thought is either past; "oooh what did I say to my friend yesterday about meeting up for a cuppa?" Or the future; "Tomorrow I will clean my car." It is never present. It may seem like you're thinking about something in the now but actually what has really happened is that you are identifying with the thought that has taken you out of the now and into a past or future moment.

With every string of thoughts there is always a chemical reaction in the body; a feeling. Sometimes the feeling comes first and then the thoughts follow, other times it's the thoughts and then very swiftly the emotion arrives. With every feeling, there are roughly 100,000 thoughts of the same vibration. This all operates like a self-fulfilling prophecy. The more we get caught up in the negative thoughts/story the more intense chemicals are released into the body. The more the body vibrates at this level the more we align with that experience and the more thoughts around that feeling arise. Unfortunately, the mind is much more pessimistic than optimistic so generally, when unconscious to this, we will identify predominantly with negative thoughts.

"People tend to dwell more on negative things than on good things. So, the mind then becomes obsessed with negative things, with judgments, guilt and anxiety produced by thoughts about the future and so on,"

Eckhart Tolle "The Power of Now."

I always like to describe us like phone masts, we are nothing more than transmitters, where the thoughts move through our experience. Thought is just energy passing through the transmitter. We see it but we are not it and as long as we don't grab it then the thought will pass through simply and easily.

It will vanish. One moment it's there the next moment it has evaporated back to where it's arisen from; consciousness. The only way the thought grows into a huge monster is when we put our attention on it, so much so, we have now gone off into a dialogue/story or a thinking process. All of which is fictitious and based in either the past or the future. When the thinking is negative, obsessive and or addicted to worry, the stress signal goes off, or even worse, we start to manifest physical symptoms such as anxiety, or depression etc.

Feelings are a fantastic gauge to tell you if you're in alignment with your truth or not. Living your truth would be:

» Basing your decisions on your intuition rather than on fear which needs to be moved through. A gut instinct happens to guide you in the right direction. Sometimes it can be unclear if it is a gut instinct or a fear. If this happens the fastest way to find your answer is to check in with your body's visceral. Close your eyes take a couple of deep breathes then ask yourself "Does saying YES make me feel alive, aligned and expansive?" Now check in with your body. Is there a light feeling or a feeling of dread? Now you know your answer. If there is a light feeling then you are listening to your intuition.

» You start intuitively listening and observing the moment. This will then allow you to see what is being presented. Sometimes that can be for you to just observe and be ok with whatever is unfolding, without labelling the experience as good or bad. Other times there may be a new decision and or a new direction to take in that moment. Or simply some truth to be spoken.
» Have you had physical injury within the last 6 months? Have you noticed feeling guilty, fearful, shameful, depressed, anxious, apathetic, angry and have pain in your body? This can be referred to as repair pain. You would only look at the suppressed/repressed emotional relationship to the pain after this time (6 months) if the pain is still there. If, after this healing time the pain seems to not want to shift, this would be a sign that there are some negative emotions held in your subconscious mind. These must be addressed before full healing can take place.

2.19. THOUGHTS AND EMOTIONS

"Thoughts are the communication language of the mind, and emotions are the feeling language of the body."

This is something I heard once from "You are the placebo: by Dr Joe Dispenza at one of his workshops in Edinburgh."

I love how this encapsulates the relationship of mind/body, thoughts and feelings. They work together, making you either feel downward spiralling and negative or upward spiralling and empowered. Thoughts and emotions have been playing a huge part in your pain. While reading these chapters, it would be great for you to watch the commentary and chatter of your mind, feelings and emotions of your body. When we learn something new or we are reminding ourselves of something we already know, we might become aware of that inner voice that tends to give a running commentary on all the new information. Take note of it while on this journey of self-empowerment, healing and letting go. Ask yourself what emotion underneath the dialogue is it triggering? For example, is there fear, hope, anger, contentment etc.

The challenge is to observe your thoughts and emotions, but only observe them, don't engage with them and continue to read the book. You can be aware of them, try not to judge them or label them as good or bad, just observe them. By the time you complete this book, you will have a clearer understanding of why I have asked you to do this.

One of the thoughts you may have is; "why can't I just skip to the end and get the tools and start implementing them now?" In order to create a lasting change, I absolutely recommend you do this small challenge. After all, you've taken the time to invest in this book with your time and finances, so why not start to change your behaviour from this moment on, and have a go at becoming the observer of your thoughts and feelings rather than engaging in them?

2.20. WHAT ARE REPRESSED EMOTIONS?

Repressed emotions are negative emotions that we unconsciously stuff down into the subconscious mind. When we experience something traumatic and or stressful the subconscious mind will repress it and almost hide it there. Unfortunately, the repressed emotions that get ignored and never acknowledged, need the most attention. Rage and anger are the most common repressed emotions, however, there can be shame, guilt, resentment, hurt and betrayal, to name a few. The reason we work to hide our emotions is that, on some level we believe vulnerability is weak and more importantly we have a fear that we may be taken advantage of. Or even worse we may be judged or rejected. However, this does come at a cost, mostly at the cost of your own health and happiness.

Then you have your "people pleasers," this characteristic is usually attributed to someone who puts everyone else first, can't say "no" and feels like they never have any time for themselves. Even if they did, they'd feel guilty for it. Whilst they are doing lots of things for others, in their subconscious mind, the emotions of resentment and rage are bubbling thick and fast. Rage gets repressed, mainly due to it not being appropriate to express at the time.

In my experience of working with people, they are generally completely unaware that rage is even there. A sign of suppressed rage is the need to blame yourself for things and to be in denial that anything is wrong. Often you feel irritated, bitter, hatred and fearful. The concerning aspect here is you may not consciously be aware that you have repressed rage but your body knows the rage is hidden in your cells which affects your health. Your brain will also sometimes purposely repress or lose the memory of an event which was so traumatic, such as rape, a severe car crash etc. in order to help you cope and survive mentally.

2.21. COMMON REPRESSED EMOTION EXAMPLES:

The emotion of envy, jealousy. This is when you find yourself comparing your life to others, it's when you feel there is a lack in your life, a lack of compassion in your world. It's when you become obsessed with what you think is missing in your life.

Have you ever found yourself in a conversation with another person who is telling you how amazing something is in their life? Meanwhile you're having a hard time with your relationship, your finances, your work etc. You walk away from the conversation and person and find yourself wishing your life was like theirs, potentially comparing it from a place of victim status "it's not fair....." Obviously not really knowing the full story of their life, but you hear what you want to hear and make a sweeping comparison in your mind. Leaving you to feel worthless, bitter, jealous and empty.

Repressed emotion results in thoughts such as; "I'm better than you" or "you'll never be as good as me." Social media is a huge trigger for envy. Seeing those perfect family days out, love and laughter and achievements. Yet the reality is you are only seeing a snap shot of the experience, the polished, intentionally chosen picture that portrays an idyllic reality. The comparing of who you are, what you've got and all the objective things in your life allows the jealousy and envy to surface into your experience. Not because these things actually make us feel this bad, but because we already have repressed and suppressed envy from past experiences that we have stuffed down into the subconscious mind. The suppressed emotion has never been dealt with and so the emotion will come back with a vengeance at any opportunity. An example of this is where you are in a newish relationship and something trivial happens. You get busy in the morning and forget to message him/her, but your partner really reacts to this. The truth is the overreaction in this case is due to past experiences, where he or she has been hurt. This then becomes filtered through the new reality.

The emotion of abandonment. No one wants to feel abandoned. Especially as connection is a key factor in human survival. So, the illusion of abandonment can make us feel we are alone. What does this lead to? This consequently makes us feel like we are not protected and therefore we feel under threat. As you know, under threat equals survival mode. If a child feels like they have been abandoned they will seek to fill the gap within. They usually do this by looking for something or someone on the outside to fill the gap. As the child matures, quite commonly they will attract unhealthy relationships with people in their life, such as abusive relationships. This is mainly because of a perceived void within. The void is love and acceptance. The characteristic behaviours of a person with repressed abandonment is one of always putting other people's needs first at the cost of their own. This results in unconscious resentment and can lead to depression.

The emotions of grief and sadness. This occurs when we don't know how to process the feeling of loss. What we tend to do with these intense emotions is push them back down into the subconscious mind. When someone loses a family member, friend, partner, child; this creates a huge amount of emotion. Of course, this is normal and is absolutely ok. However, once the funeral is over there is an expectation to return back to life, which is what we do. But emotion still keeps rising up and we begin to feel bad for still feeling down so we suppress our feelings of grief. We believe we have to be strong for others or perhaps that it's time to get back on with life regardless of how we actually feel. The consequence of this is, through default, we suppress joy. How this happens is by denying what you need. You compromise, which comes at a cost, lost joy. Grieving is a natural part of letting go and it is also ok to grieve. However, when we suppress emotions such as grief and sadness it will inevitably try its hardest to surface until dealt with. This can have the appearance of someone who suffers with low mood, mood swings and or anxiety. When really it is an emotion which wants to be headed on and let go of. Stuffing it back down, resisting it and therefore suppressing it is hard work, exhausting and if not dealt with, will have a negative impact on a person's health and life.

The emotions of anger and rage. Repressed anger happens when our basic human needs are not being met. Basic needs, to feel safe, connected, have food, warmth and a roof over our heads, a purpose and love. When these are challenged, it will anger us. A great example of this is when we are misunderstood by someone who may not have understood all the details. Because they don't have the full picture you feel threatened and instantly feel anger. It is the egoic part of your mind which is feeling misunderstood. Anger always surfaces when there is any form of bullying. Anger also becomes repressed when we simply learn that expressing it is not acceptable. People pleasers are great at repressing anger, as they repeatedly carry on putting other people's needs before their own. Said another way, it is when you feel too vulnerable to express how you really feel. You may notice in your own past behaviour that it feels so much easier to express boundaries once you are feeling upset. Think of a time when you finally got angry and only then did you find yourself saying what needed to be said. Unfortunately, setting boundaries via anger is an unhealthy method. It is the negative or destructive energy that is powering the shift.

The emotion resentment. I always find this emotion so fascinating because most people that have resentment suppressed in their subconscious have no idea that they feel resentful. They have mastered the art of doing things for others from a place of hidden resentment. Once the person is aware that they feel resentful, it allows them to become a pillar of strength, and express boundaries. Resentful people are usually not great at boundary setting and can't say "no." Therefore, they carry deep seated resentment. This can be married up with guilt at times. They say yes because they feel guilty yet harbour resentment for not saying no.

The emotion of fear. With real-time fear, we create a "fight or flight" response. However, when we repress fear it can literally immobilise us. The body goes into freeze mode. Fear paralyses us. This is the natural response to trauma as the brain will always seek to keep you alive. It does this by protecting you. However, fear is a symptom of trauma.

The emotions of shame and guilt. Shame and guilt are prevalent in our society. How many of us can hold our hand up and say we've carried guilt based on what we think others may be thinking about us, letting people down and not being able to say no? Yet again we are prepared to carry resentment, often the resentment is unconscious. Not obvious until we ask ourselves "am

I truly happy with saying no." Then shame creeps in when we create an unrealistic high expectation for ourselves. We don't feel worthy. This can also manifest when a person who is influential in your life gives you the impression that setting boundaries are selfish. You learn that poor boundaries are equal to love and acceptance.

Shame: Is this unpleasant emotion which leaves you feeling self-conscious. It is typically associated with feelings of distress, mistrust, powerlessness, and worthlessness.

Guilt: Guilt is said to be the greatest destroyer of emotional energy. Guilt sucks your energy dry, it leaves you feeling bad. A sense of dread that you should have done something differently.

2.22. WHAT ARE SUPPRESSED EMOTIONS?

To suppress is to consciously (as opposed to repressed being when it happens without your knowing) stuff negative emotion down into your subconscious mind. To avoid them as you do not really know what to do with them. Examples of this are: anger, grief, sadness, shame, apathy, fear etc. We adopt compulsive behaviours, bad habits, and disruptive ways to feel better. The most common trait of suppressed emotion is projection, a defence mechanism around dealing with uncomfortable negative emotions. This is where you project your emotions onto the outside. Usually a person, situation or thing.

I have to say I find this so incredibly fascinating. I know I've done this lots throughout my own life, taken disturbing emotions and traits about myself and projected them onto someone else, believing at that moment that he or she was the person with the problem. We only project uncomfortable feelings. This is when we end up making that person we have projected the feelings and traits onto, our enemy. That's because the feeling of fear, anger or guilt can be so intense that the only way to deal with it is to reflect it away from ourselves and onto someone else, aka the blame culture.

You would know if you have suppressed/repressed emotions in your subconscious because those who have are more likely to feel irritated by being asked how you feel about something or someone. In fact, the question makes you feel blank, angry, annoyed, speechless, powerless and confused. It almost feels like you are experiencing a violation of your privacy.

The body is a direct reflection of your subconscious mind. The metaphysical anatomy explains that each part of the body is linked to an emotional cause. When it comes to pain, illness and disease, depending on where it is manifesting in your body would depend on the emotional blockage in the subconscious mind. Your body is communicating to you that there is something somewhere in your life that doesn't align with your absolute truth or what you truly desire. Usually, in my experience, there is a repressed or suppressed emotion that needs to be let go of, and, potentially a change in your environment to be made. Maybe a change of relationship to your thinking mind (as in what are you focusing on, obsessing about or thinking about) and the outside world but most importantly there is a significant change that needs to be made in your behaviour which isn't serving you anymore. I don't mean in an attitude of behaviour, rather an unconscious behaviour that is on repeat.

Let's identify if you have REPRESSED/SUPPRESSED EMOTIONS?

If you are human and have ever experienced anything stressful in your life you will have suppressed or repressed emotions in your subconscious mind. But here are some great questions to ask yourself to confirm this. While answering the following, be as truthful as possible. Tick the boxes if relevant, there may be more than one.

» Do I find it impossible to open up and share my true feelings with people?

» Would I rather say nothing than reveal what I am truly feeling?
» Do I believe that anger and sadness are emotions that are not acceptable, especially when I see it in other people's behaviour?
» Do I knowingly do my best to cover anger and sadness up?
» Do I see myself as "laid back" and if we were to talk about anger or stress would I say to you "I'm one of those lucky people, I don't get stressed or feel anger very often if ever" Perhaps you will say; "I don't feel stressed"
» Do I dislike or avoid confrontation?
» Do I struggle with knowing what I am feeling?
» Do I portray many escape behaviours, like binge eating, binge drinking, binge drugs, binge shopping, oversleeping, gossiping, gambling, jumping from relationship to relationship?
» Can I remember the last time I cried? It's not something I feel I need to do?
» Do I feel really uncomfortable around emotionally charged people, perhaps it makes me feel very awkward?
» Do I have a tendency to overreact when I get angry, am I only seeing that this is what I do as I read this question to myself now?
» Do I notice I don't want to stop the negative thoughts?
» Am I self-critical (all the time)?

- » Do I gossip and talk about other people with ease?
- » Do I always need to be in control, I don't like not being in control, the idea freaks me out?

2.23. THE MIND AND THE EGO

Why is it sometimes so difficult to do the smallest things? Even taking the simplest actions that we know will improve our lives seems impossible. Why? The mind has been designed to STOP you at all costs doing anything that may be threatening to you. Sometimes this 'stopping' can manifest in your experience like you have lost your mojo or your motivation has disappeared. The truth is; the way your mind has been wired up is to not do things that cause discomfort, fear or difficulty. In fact, our brains have been designed to protect us from all of the above. The brain is trying to keep us alive at all times. However, in order for you to become the best version of yourself at work or with family, friends and life in general, you will have to do something new from time to time. You may have a perceived feeling of this being difficult, often because we have to leave our comfort zone to learn something new.

We may not have any control over what is being presented to us in life. However, there are three things that we do have control over:

- The meaning we give something
- The attention we give something
- The decisions we make

Let me expand on these.

Meaning: The meaning we give something - look at the activity, person or thing you are about to embark on, have you wrapped fear, uncertainty or dread to the outcome? Does the meaning need updating?

Attention: The attention we give something. This could be time, money, energy etc but always stick to one rule; if you're going to do something well then give it 100%. There is no room for 99% effort.

Finally: The decision you make. You are making decisions all day long whether you are aware of it or not. The fact you are reading this book is a decision you made. Even when you make the decision to not make a decision you are making a decision! So, start consciously making decisions and see how quickly life changes for the better.

Dr Joe Dispenza mentions in all his publications Evolve your brain "the mind is the brain in action." The brain may have tripled in size over the past seven million years, however as mentioned before, it still operates with similar traits to that of a caveman. The blueprint of the body has stayed the same even though humans and their living style has completely shifted. Back then, the ego helped protect humans, as it still does today. However, the threats which we face today are nothing like they were. The ego mind would relentlessly look for dilemmas and obstacles, such as, "Watch out, there is a huge scary animal coming toward you and it looks hungry. Run now!"

The egoic mind is still continually looking for potential life-threatening problems. If you're not aware that the egoic mind is NOT who you are, then it can sound very convincing. It is that voice, that inner commentary, that sometimes sounds like you, sometimes it morphs into a parent or a teacher or a friend's voice. It's literally like having that person on your shoulders continuously, running a narrative. Its main role is to look for problems so that it can keep your body safe and you alive. I bet you have heard the phrase; "get the monkey off your back......"

The ego mind is the aspect of every human being that can seem like the enemy when you have no awareness of its traits. Without this awareness, it can throw you into living your life on red alert; taking you off into future forecasting, often using your imagination in a negative way, leaving you feeling like there's a constant problem on the horizon - even if life is good! A negative thought questions "why is everything going well, it's bound to stop and crumble soon?" The ego is never happy or content and is ruthless in its gloomy commentary and throws up these thoughts.

A great question to ask yourself, to see if you're filtering through ego (sometimes best thought of as "the illusion") is: In this moment, do I feel inferior or superior to others? If the answer is "yes" to either then you are definitely running your experience through ego! The ego mind lives in the past or it lives in the future. It is not present. It's wrapped in thought and negative emotions. It will find a past experience, it could be something that you've witnessed, it might be something you've seen on TV or even heard, it might not even be your story, it might be somebody else's - but the ego mind grabs evidence, then projects it into a future moment and makes it seem about a hundred times worse. It's always coming from a state of fear.

Low vibrational emotions are wrapped around fear and ego. It tends to say "you can't do something" over "you're amazing, you can do this." Both are actually ego, however since ego is pessimistic by nature it generally will tell you the "can't" version. The ego mind is actually not the villain, but unless you are aware of how it works; unless you know what it is; it becomes, for most people, their nemesis! They don't realise that it's not who they ARE. It is 100% judgmental. It is negative, critical, and it is harsh.

For me, it's that voice that I was trying to escape fifteen years ago, and I didn't realise it wasn't who I was. The more stressed you become, the louder and more intense it gets.

"The ego is the false self - born out of fear and defensiveness,"

John O'Donohue.

The ego shows up in a number of ways, often disguised. Have you ever found yourself in an argument feeling very driven to be right, because winning is very important to you in that moment? The stubbornness takes over, the need to be rigorous? Right? moves in and you're consumed in getting your point over at all costs? Or perhaps you can you see that you often have unrealistic goals which leads to you spending most of your life beating yourself up over not achieving them? Such as "I will start this diet and lose a stone in 10 days." Yet by Wednesday you are eating sugar, drinking wine and had pizza for supper, so again you feel dreadful and guilty so tell yourself you will start again on Monday. A never-ending cycle that goes on and on. The extreme of the diet is too much and only leads to self-sabotage and beating yourself up when you seemingly fail yet again. Maybe you've experienced jealousy especially when you see or hear someone is happy or heaven forbid, they are doing well in life? The feeling is again, one of "it's not fair." Do you find that you can talk about yourself all day long, yet regrettably, you're so wrapped up in yourself it doesn't enter your conscious awareness to ask how anyone else is doing? Do you have a tendency to blame others when things don't go your way, looking outwards at the world for excuses to make yourself feel better? Looking at parents to blame for your misfortunes as an adult, ex-partners for a poor settlement, friends who seemingly don't do what you think they should do for you? Are you addicted to gossiping and will harness any opportunity to speak in great detail about your opinion on someone else's life, to the point that you're happy to compare yourself to those you believe are better and or worse than you? If the answer is "yes" to any of the above then you are in your ego! If you're saying "yikes" right about now don't worry, we have all done some, if not all of the above. This is definitely not about humiliating you to get your attention, it's about bringing awareness to behaviours that do not serve you.

A Course In Miracles by Helen Schucman says that "the ego is suspicious at best and vicious at worst." I can see that. The other thing about the egoic mind is the contrast. When we are born, we are born into a state of unconditional love, total perfection, which is our natural birth right. The beautiful thing about being a human being is that we get to experience a contrast of opposites. We have positive/negative, we have black/white, we have night/day. We also have movement and stillness. It is this contrast that sets us apart from all other creatures and is the bedrock of our path to enlightenment.

When we are aware enough to realise, we are not our mind - we have a choice! To come back and rest into our birth right state of total bliss, joy and happiness. The present moment. The present moment is where you are no longer identified with thought. You are aware of thought moving through your experience yet you consciously choose to be still in the moment, observing your mind and thought. It is here where healing, truth, expansion, possibility, potential and unconditional love exist. Without that contrast, you would not know that you're actually bathing in bliss and joy because you wouldn't know what suffering is.

It's only the perception of our ego that makes it "negative," I try not to judge the ego as negative now and to just observe it with curiosity as it does what it does. When you are not aware of it - then you will be run by it convinced by the things it tells you, often believing that there are problems, potential disasters about to occur with a constant worry about all sorts of things going wrong. With awareness, you can start to separate from the ego and start to observe it rather than believing what it is saying.

I think one of the biggest and most profound breakthroughs that I've had on this journey is that "awareness always precedes all change." Only when we become aware of our mind and our body and who we are as a human being - not human doing - do we get our power back and the choice to do something different.

2.24. WHAT IS EGO – RECAP

» It doesn't know anything about reality. It runs from programming - the only aspect of you that knows reality is consciousness.
» It's a software programme that is designed to give feedback.
» Ego gathers data that it's observing then takes that data and makes it personal.
» It doesn't really exist, it is a mind-made programme, a software programme of the mind.

The ego is NOT:

» Intuition, or
» Instinct, or
» Intentions

The ego is a mechanism that comments on your intuition, instinct or intentions. It is inherently selfish by nature. Consciousness is infinite - in order for it to experience itself, it has to project the illusion of being infinite. The body and your life are your objective experience and a direct reflection of your subconscious mind. The fastest way to find out if something is holding you back is to have a look at your body and your objective life and ask yourself a simple question;

What in my life is not in alignment with my truth? To explain this; being in alignment with your truth is to create for your greater good, to expand and to avoid being caught listening to your egoic mind. The nomenclature surrounding the F.A.M. was born out of this principal, being free from constraints of the mind and in alignment with what serves you best. Freedom Alignment! It's also a method!

Perhaps, you have some physical pain. Or you are carrying some extra pounds in weight. Maybe you have a dislike for your body or parts of it. There is always a neighbour that is angry at you; perhaps your relationships are difficult and challenging. Maybe life feels stressful or hard. Perhaps you feel like you have never got any money, maybe your career is not right, potentially you are just unhappy. Anything that is not an experience of prosperity, health and abundance is a sure sign to tell you that there are some subconscious limiting beliefs and suppressed/repressed emotions in your subconscious mind. The best thing you can do is take the time to write a list of the things right now that you feel are out of alignment.

2.25. THE CONSCIOUS MIND

The Conscious mind makes up 5% of your brain, and it is the aspect of your mind which is the visionary, conceptual and ideas part of the brain. It learns in a completely different way to the subconscious mind. The conscious mind could pick this book up, read it and decide that changes need to be made in your life now. The intentions will be pure and valid, the big problem here is that if your subconscious mind is not in alignment to that particular foresight, idea or vision, it will sabotage it. This is because the subconscious mind is 30,000 times more powerful than the conscious mind. It is why it is pointless trying to make changes from the outside. Change is an inside job; only when we identify the conflict and thus make the conscious changes will the conscious and subconscious mind be able to align with your dreams and visions. It is then that anything is possible.

Traits of the conscious mind

» It will discriminate
» It will choose
» It will analyse
» It will invent
» It will judge

» It will criticise
» It will plan

2.26. THE SUBCONSCIOUS MIND

I find this part of the mind beyond fascinating as, without this knowledge, you could live your life going round and round in a circle of madness. With this information, you can see now, how and what has been the driving force of your choices. The power of having the following information is that you can choose to live life with much more fluidity and joy rather than seriousness and stress. Firstly, you must know that the subconscious mind is a recording of your entire existence. Yes, that is right; everything you have ever experienced has been noted down. From being in the womb in the third trimester, you have been recording and observing, tasting, looking and listening. Once born, you observe through your senses. You see those around you, like your parents, teachers, siblings, your culture, your town, your family, your friends, your world. You observe, and you download other people's ways, traits, behaviours and beliefs like programmes. This is necessary for the first seven years of your life, to give you the knowledge of how to fit into society, and survive. The subconscious mind lives in the past, filtering past experiences into your now, it colours your reality with your beliefs so we don't see things as they are only how we believe them to be. The subconscious mind is a pessimist; the way it works is like a programme which has been set to protect you and therefore will do whatever it takes to keep you in your comfort zone. If you do not consciously clear out the limiting beliefs and suppressed emotions, it will eventually manifest as pain or illness in the body and your life.

2.27. WHAT SHAPES YOUR SUBCONSCIOUS MIND?

Everything: Taste, vision, hearing, touch, smell and noise! It's all downloaded and recorded.

By the time a child gets to secondary school they will have been exposed, on average, to 8,000 simulated murders on T.V. All these images sink into the child's subconscious mind. Don't be fooled by cartoons from Hollywood either. In the most critical years of developmental where a child needs to learn compassion and love, instead, we see our children subjected to violent stories subliminally through listening to radio, T.V. and what appear to be innocent films. You have to remember a child's mind is like a sponge.

2.28. RULES OF THE SUBCONSCIOUS MIND

» Your subconscious mind likes to do as little as possible.
» All emotions live in the subconscious mind.

- They are attached to memories and experiences.
- Emotions drive all of our decisions.
- Humans will unconsciously do whatever it takes to move from emotions of pain to pleasure.
- Your subconscious mind doesn't recognise negativity at first. If you tell yourself "DON'T think of a pink cow," it will firstly picture the pink cow then process the command. Have you ever wondered why a child, when told "Don't touch!" the first thing they do is touch it. It's because he/she thinks that that is what you are asking them to do initially.
- The subconscious mind runs many bodily functions so that we don't have to remember to do it ourselves, such as breathing, blood pumping around the body and digestion. (It is so clever!).
- We filter millions of bits of information that are received every second through the subconscious mind so that your conscious mind only has to pay attention to relevant information.
- The conscious mind can only process seven pieces of information at the same time.
- Your subconscious mind is always programmed to want more; it's never satisfied which is a trap and an illusion that you must watch out for. It is why most people are not satisfied. They are always searching for more, taking themselves out of the present moment and into a future one,

basing happiness on a time and place that's not now.

» Your habits reflect the quality of your life, and an addiction is a behavioural pattern stored in your subconscious mind. It takes 21 days to create a new habit.
» Your subconscious mind is like a small child or obedient servant; it wants, and only follows, directly from the conscious mind. However, you should be aware of the language you choose to use as the subconscious mind follows strict orders. If you say "I don't touch that hot plate" then your subconscious mind will hear you want to be fat. On the flip side when you know how it works you can also do the opposite. Put your attention on what you do want. Almost like the phrase "fake it 'til you make it." You tell yourself you can do something. Remember the subconscious mind doesn't understand negativity.

"Whatever we plant in our subconscious mind and nourish with repetition and emotion will one day become a reality"

Earl Nightingale

2.29. THE BODY

There is nothing to work out; if you are disconnected from your truth, the body will send you a message through emotional, physical or mental pain. Your muscles are what give you the flexibility to move and have the strength to get on with life. They are also where you hold all of your energy. Trauma shows up in the muscles and causes them to weaken and in some cases, lock up. Carl Georgii coined the term "kinesiology" in 1854 and perfectly explained this process:

"Kinesiology is a non-invasive holistic energy therapy, combining the ancient principles of Traditional Chinese Medicine (TCM) with modern muscle monitoring techniques. Kinesiology uses muscle-testing techniques to gain an insight into the areas of stress and imbalance within the energy system. It is based upon the premise that any issues within an energy system will eventually be reflected in the body."

Therapy directory, kinesiology

Translated, this is a method to measure and identify imbalances in the body's chemical, structural and emotional energy. David Hawkins spoke a lot about this method due to his massive amount of work and research around the power of kinesiology. The answers are always within us. Isn't it crazy that this is often one of the last places people go to find health? The outside world is consciousness objectified. Consciousness being the cause and the effect (the substance) of the world you experience. Our reality has two parts; the conscious and subconscious and the relationship between these two areas is significant.

The subconscious mind has been busy recording your entire life. It therefore files away memories, suppressed emotion, experiences, and perspectives like a computer programme. All this information is stored away and kept on file. We are not always conscious of it. However, muscle testing allows you to access this information. A little bit like that moment you forgot your P.I.N. for your bank card. You rack your brain, and nothing happens. Then you go to the hole in the wall to get some money out and boom somehow your fingers know the pin. The body has become the mind and programmed to punch in a sequence of numbers without thinking about it. The body has accessed information from the subconscious mind.

2.30. THE MIND/BODY CONNECTION

Thoughts are the functions of the mind and emotions are the chemistry of the body. They work alongside each other and depending on where you put your attention first; then the other will be triggered.

An example of this came up whilst I wrote this book, a lady came to my door, she looked dishevelled, and her voice shaky. The first words that left her mouth were: "can you tell me why you would park your car with the wheel over the white line?" She had a fair point; it was ever so slightly over the white line. She then went on to say she can't get her car out and quipped some unrepeatable expletives. Interestingly, in the moment of her venting, her previous days/weeks/ life problems were what threw these words at me, I stood and listened. Slightly taken back by her final comments, I grabbed my car keys and moved my car to keep the peace, perhaps in this moment, I became a massive people pleaser.

I share this for two reasons, firstly: the tone of her voice and the shakiness in her tones suggested that she had been in her mind before getting to me. It had already created a chemical reaction in her physiology. Secondly, the mirror effect was in full play here. She thought she was angry with me but the truth is that the woman was experiencing energy she labelled as anger. The car was stuck out and she attached the emotion to it through projection, unconsciously admittedly. She had no clue what she was doing. She was acting from a feeling that was so strong it drove her to knock on my door and say what she had to say to move her from pain to pleasure. As in all interactions, there was, of course, something in it for me too.

2.31. WHAT IS A NEED?

Abraham Maslow created a theory called Maslow's Hierarchy of Needs. These needs included; physiological, safety, love and belonging, esteem, and self-actualisation. As our needs are met , our motivation increases as a human. It creates growth in a person. Happiness is the definition of a human progressing continually. When we feel like we are developing, there is a real sense of purpose and contentment. I have a theory (not proven, just an intuitive hunch) that common illnesses such as Parkinson's Disease sets in when an active person's functions stop both mentally and physically. It's like the brain and body become stagnant and so literally like inactive water, toxicity sets in, the flow becomes stuck, and slowly the mind starts to switch off.

What the different types of "needs" mean

» **Physiological** - the things we need for human survival such as air, sleep, food, sex, clothing, drink, shelter and warmth. If these basic needs are not met, a human cannot function.

» **Safety** - freedom from fear, protection, security, law and stability.

» **Love and belongingness** - this is more of a social need and involves feeling the need for connection with another which always results in a person being more motivated. Healthy relationships evoke happiness, motivation and joy. We are social, tribal creatures and need human connection.

» **Esteem** - this should be broken into two. Firstly - esteem for oneself (how you see yourself). Secondly - the recognition from another. Recognition is the number one motivator in a human.
» **Self-actualisation** - reaching your potential, self-fulfilment, going inwards, personal growth. Your desire to become the best version of yourself through living your best life!

Tony Robbins has taken Maslow's hierarchy of needs and put his slant on it. He says we all have six human needs that are important for harmony. The main human drivers of behaviour seemingly all point to the number one need; connection – all humans must feel connection (love), or we die.

Tony Robbins, 6 Basic Needs:

1. **Certainty:** Assurance you can avoid pain and gain pleasure. The need for safety and security about your future.
2. **Uncertainty/variety:** The need for the unknown, change, new stimuli.
3. **Significance:** Feeling unique, important, special or needed - a desire to be heard, seen or listened to.

4. **Connection/Love:** A strong feeling of closeness or union with someone or something.
5. **Growth:** An expansion of capacity, capability or understanding.
6. **Contribution:** A sense of service and focus on helping, giving to and supporting others. "The secret to living is giving!" Tony Robbins

The long and short of it, is that humans are greatly influenced by their conscious or unconscious desire to have their needs met. Needs are subjective - how one person sees a need can be different from another because of their perception, life experience and programming. These can be affected by our personal values too. When we feel negative feelings, they are your internal alarm bell showing you that your needs are NOT being met. Some examples of these feelings can be, anger, annoyance, bitterness, boredom, confusion, depression, embarrassment and guilt to name a few.

2.32. WHAT IS A VALUE?

A value is a conscious choice to act in a particular manner to meet your own needs. Once you know what your core values are, it becomes much easier to meet them. Values are the principles that give our lives meaning and allow us to persevere through adversity, according to psychologist Barb Markway and Celia

Ample. Values influence our behaviour too and fulfilment comes from aligning with our core values.

Unfortunately, when we do not live our lives according to what is truly important to us, we often find ourselves behaving in ways to numb the negative thoughts and emotions that this causes, such as drink, drugs, shopping, spending money we don't have, obsessing, procrastinating, gossiping, judging etc. These are distraction techniques. We are experts at distracting ourselves from our feelings. However, knowing what your core values are will change your life. This is an integral aspect of the Freedom Alignment Method. Go to the "values exercise" section later in the book to find out what your core values are.

3. CHAPTER THREE: THE FREEDOM ALIGNMENT METHOD (F.A.M.)

The Freedom Alignment Method (F.A.M.) is a technique that has taken more than 15 years to create. The F.A.M. addresses the direct cause of emotional, physical and mental pain, illness, disease or anxiety and depression. It does this by accessing the root instigator; our emotions. As mentioned above, the brain is programmed to protect and keep us alive so it makes unconscious decisions to support our wellbeing. In the event of a stressful experience and if the mind thinks it can't cope, it will take the intense emotion that has been created such as anger, shame, guilt or fear and suppress it into the subconscious mind. The F.A.M. works at uncovering or exposing these repressed and suppressed emotions and setting them free, using a myriad of different mental tools and exercises thus allowing us to live our best life, free from anxiety and stress.

3.1. HOW DOES THE FREEDOM ALIGNMENT METHOD WORK?

The F.A.M. works on the following principles, philosophies and rules.

» We learn through society to block and avoid our negative emotions. F.A.M. helps you identify your blocks and uncovers the suppressed/repressed emotions.

- Awareness precedes all change. It is essential to not only know this but to use this principal in every aspect of life, becoming aware of something, anything, is the fundamental first learning in order to change it.
- We create negative beliefs around the meaning we give to intense emotions such as guilt, shame, anger etc.
- We learn from a young age that expressing "negative" emotions is a bad thing, so we suppress the feeling instead.
- When we don't feel our emotions. Our emotions end up feeling us.
- Not addressing emotions that arise in our experience ultimately affects our mental and physical health.
- Suppressed emotions cut off the blood flow and constrict blood vessels and create blockages in the body. These eventually cause physical pain.
- We are ruled by our emotions, generally unconsciously - only with awareness can change be made.
- Acknowledgement of what you're experiencing regarding your emotions is the first step to self-empowerment.
- The more emotionally conflicted a person feels, the more anxiety they will feel. Period.

- Negative emotions signal to the body, the body then reacts with the stress hormone as it believes you are under threat.
- One of the reasons why emotions are essential is that they are the indicator to show whether you are in or out of alignment or homeostasis (health).
- A recurring negative emotion is also a sign that suppressed emotion is rising from the subconscious and is ready to be released. The natural tendency of a human (when unconscious to this) is to stuff the emotion back down into the subconscious mind immediately. So, the cycle continues.
- We have no control over the emotions that are triggered; however, we do have complete control over perspective, meaning and what actions we take as we address the moment.
- We live in a culture of escapism when really what is needed is to unlearn our old habits of avoidance so we can relearn how not to fear what is being presented.
- It is vital to change our relationship to any negative emotion by learning to experience all feelings without judgement.
- When labelling is removed, what is left is an experience of energy which is neither good nor bad; it just is. To experience that is to allow the feeling and then the feeling can be freed.

- » Only then can an actual letting go process be activated and from this place change and alignment of homeostasis can and does take place.
- » Your mind controls your body through identification to thoughts and feelings.
- » Whatever is held in the mind will always reflect itself in the body.
- » The body is not who you are.
- » The mind is the brain in action. The brain is the physical substance and the mind is the conscious product of those firing neurones. The mind is not confined to the size of your skull or body. David Hawkins described it as "the seat of consciousness." It is what makes you feel alive. (I love this).
- » Watch the words you use and the words you are thinking as these are key to keeping you trapped in old ways and habits. When you wake up to this unconscious dialogue, you can change your settings. In other words, you can stop sabotaging your existence by taking your focus away from lack, fear and worry and start placing your attention on wealth, health, joy and peace. The fastest way to experience these things is to master the art of living in the "NOW."
- » Let go of the resistance always; this is your only job if I am honest.

- » Don't give your physical pain a label; let it go by shifting from resisting the pain to allowing it – always. In other words; let go of wanting it to go away.
- » Suppressed/repressed negative feelings can cause physical and mental pain and illnesses.
- » Suppressed/repressed emotions, habits, and feelings cause thoughts.
- » The possibility of becoming the observer of your thoughts and emotions must be understood. You have been resisting or stuffing down these feelings your entire life. Let them be FELT and DEALT!
- » Strong feelings that keep recurring in your experience have one meaning; there is more to let go of, and that's ok.
- » Sometimes the first thing you must surrender/let go of is the feeling of guilt. It is because you have an unconscious belief or suppressed emotion that by letting this go, you are doing something wrong.
- » Guess what? Negative feelings aren't who you are.
- » It is not about focusing on changing your thoughts - it's about being ok with thoughts yet not going off into thinking.
- » "Feel, deal & dump" (see the F.A.M. Feel, deal & dump exercise) rather than "resist and persist."

- Stop focusing and verbalising your victim story - your mind and body are listening.
- Understand; your body knows how to heal; the powerhouse of your body protects you. Technically it is part of your immune system, it's called your immunoglobulin A (IGA). These Protection Protein Antibodies are so advanced and intelligent they will outweigh any vaccination. The only time they become switched off is when your body is under continual stress. Otherwise, the body is an incredible piece of kit; it just needs your support in letting go of the blocks (suppressed/repressed emotion) so that it can do its job.
- Everything is happening for our greater good - the pain, illness, disease? It's your teacher. What is it trying to show you? What do you need to let go of, see and or become?
- Your body is the chemist so let it do its job.
- To fully let go, we must accept and then surrender any secondary gains to the illness, pain and or behaviour - a bitter pill to swallow for many of us but necessary to align with your health.
- Let go of the desire to control the outcome of your life. Some pain and illness may disappear within days/weeks; others may take longer. You have to be ok with not being ok. Or you will return to resistance, and this will keep you trapped in pain.

3.2. FREEDOM ALIGNMENT METHOD EXERCISES

The Four-Step Process of the Freedom Alignment Method.

1. F.A.M. AWARENESS - Bring awareness to your thoughts and feelings.
2. F.A.M. METAPHYSICAL ANATOMY - Where in the body is my pain?
3. F.A.M. ACTION - Release the feelings and emotions around your pain.
4. F.A.M. ANTIDOTE - Transcend into a state of wellbeing and alignment.

3.3. HOW TO USE THIS SECTION

To get the best results, you need to follow the process below. Sometimes there is more to let go of than at other times. Therefore, you may have to repeat the process more than once. However, as long as you follow the process, you will get the results.

Firstly, make sure you have paper and pen, you are sitting comfortably and you have the time to do this process without distraction. Set yourself 30 minutes.

Have an open mind. Focus only on the question or statement that you want to work with. Do your best to answer the question without overthinking it. In other words, take pen to paper and just write whatever is there to write.

Try not to analyse any of it; just write and trust. Your mind will try and jump in at times. Just come back to the question and keep on writing until there is nothing flowing from your pen. Remember you can't get this wrong. Whatever comes up is correct in that moment.

3.4. HEART & MIND CONNECTION EXERCISE

This process allows you to stay anchored in the present moment and tap into your intuition, to listen to what your body is saying. It will enable you to align with your potential and empower you to be the best you can be. You may need to do this for each question at first but as you become used to the practice, you will find it easier to make the connection between your heart and mind.

Close your eyes and get comfortable. Feet placed on the ground and body relaxed. Take three deep breaths then on each out breath visualise that you are releasing the stresses of the day from the cells of your body, with ease.

On your fourth breath, I would now like you to imagine that you are taking your mind on a journey to the back of your throat. The throat has a slide, which the mind is going to slide down.

Your mind is sliding down the back of the throat and joining the heart. Your heart and mind are now connected. Now, gently open your eyes to answer the questions below. Between each question come back to the mind and heart connection. Then move onto the next question.

3.5. AWARENESS – BRINGING AWARENESS TO YOUR THOUGHTS AND FEELINGS

Awareness precedes all change - this powerhouse of a statement is the catalyst to your success. Without awareness of what is going on in your experience it will be impossible to heal. So, follow the questions below to guide you through the F.A.M process and collect all the relevant information to continue your journey of healing.

Identify where the physical, emotional or mental pain is. Where is the pain in your body, mind or experience? (Physical, emotional and or mental). There may be more than one thing going on, that's ok - write it all down.

- Where in the body is my pain?
- When did the pain begin?

- » Specifically - What stress was in my life at the time or just before the time the pain began?

Think about this: What was going on at the time, emotionally and mentally in both a subjective and objective sense? Take time to answer this - sometimes the knee-jerk reaction to this question is to say "nothing." Take each area of your life and break it down into work, relationships, finance, family, children, holidays, self-development, education, purpose, progression, home etc. Ask yourself what stresses were going on in these areas of your life? What stresses did you focus on in your mind around the time the pain began? Did you worry? Were you catastrophising a future outcome? Overthinking? Concerned what others may think? Focusing on "what if's?"

Concentrate now on Physical Pain

Mark each pain out of 10. (1 = low and 10 = high)

Don't overthink this just put the first number that comes up into your awareness and trust that's right.

- » Joint pain
- » Chronic back pain
- » Asthma and hay fever
- » Headaches and migraines
- » Chest pain
- » Poor sleep
- » Menstruation problems

» Fibromyalgia
» Addictive behaviour
» Sleep issues/Insomnia
» Anxiety & depression
» Skin problems (acne, psoriasis)
» Irritable Bowel Syndrome (I.B.S.)
» Diarrhoea, bloating, constipation
» High blood pressure
» Other

Do this for 2 minutes every day. At the end of meditation practice is best, but if you don't meditate, then you can still do it. Keep this as your focus, feeling every time your mind tries to convert you back into your old way of thinking.

It's time to see that the body is nothing more than a direct reflection of the subconscious mind. Reflecting and showing you that it is time to let go of whatever suppressed emotion(s) you are holding onto so that you can return to balance. A vital point to make is that the pain wouldn't be showing up if you weren't ready to make this change.

What next?

The only thing you need to do is "let go" of the repressed emotion. Surrender the feeling! When you surrender the repressed emotion/feeling, it starts to dissolve very quickly. The only reason it may not disappear completely is that there is more to let go of. You can be gentle with yourself over this process as you've spent a lifetime consciously and or unconsciously "stuffing" your feelings into your subconscious mind.

"Shame is the most powerful, master emotion. It's the fear that we're not good enough." Brene Brown - The Power of Vulnerability

Am I experiencing emotional/mental pain?

It is crucial here to write out the answers to the questions asked below. The questions are designed to allow you to get to the core cause of your pain. Take your time and be gentle with yourself. Some of the questions will likely feel hard to answer but trust your intuition.

Your heart and mind know your truth. Also, if a question does not feel applicable move on to the next.

» Do you feel that someone has harmed you (emotionally, mentally, physically, spiritually) in your life? Or continues to hurt you?
» If so, who is this person and how does this person make you feel?
» Do you spend your life obsessing over things or people? If so, what do you obsess over?
» Does the obsession feel like you can't change it?

- Which of the following do you recognise experiencing? Resentment, out of control grief, anger or another?
- Are you living the life you want? Be honest, and if not, why not? What stops you?
- Are you living in the past?
- What emotions are you trying to suppress? If you are not sure, then follow the Freedom Alignment Method "Feel, Deal and Dump" exercise.
- Do you feel angry for allowing yourself to get into a place of feeling disempowered by a seemingly influential person? Yes or no?
- If yes, who is the person and why? How does this make you feel?
- Do you have a fear of the unknown?
- What are you doing that you don't want to do? (work, relationships, finances, health, friendships etc).
- Has life stopped being joyful? If so, why has it?

Now you have your list. This is a list of experiences that you identified that you may have suppressed or repressed into your subconscious mind. Put this list down onto paper, you will be using it later on in the book.

I really want to highlight a crucial learning here. This is a key moment of the healing process and is the first step of the Freedom Alignment Method. As mentioned before, AWARENESS precedes all change. Now we need to take this to the next level and look at the mind-body connection.

3.5.1. F.A.M. METAPHYSICAL ANATOMY – WHERE IN THE BODY IS MY PAIN?

The Metaphysical Anatomy represents the connection between mind and body and is primarily based upon the principle of, “as above so below, as within so without.” Hermes Trismegistus. This means as something happens, on a particular level of reality, it also happens on an another. In terms of the body and mind, it describes the link between the health of your body and the health of your environment, relationship, perspective, attitude, habits, beliefs and world? The human being is a combination of mind, body, spirit and emotions. All these areas interact with each other and influence who we are and how we feel.

What we experience in one area of your life will inevitably affect all areas of life. You only have to look at your life today and see how each stress affects different areas of your life. Each bodily symptom from illness or injury has a story to tell you about yourself and your life. It is always the signpost trying to get your attention to say there is something here you need to address, change or let go of. Only then can the healing take place.

So, what is your body telling you?

Your body is a reflection of your subconscious mind. Whatever shows up in the body is a reflection of what is going on in the outside world, is an opportunity to make change – particularly if the body is presenting with pain and discomfort and is just an opportunity (if you don't like it) to see and let go of something. It is the dance of life. These two areas become the road map to change. As we allow the change to happen, our "needs" align, and we become more complete, fulfilled. Your job is to be open to that change with no attachment to how it may unfold. In my experience, this is where a higher level of peace exists.

3.5.2. METAPHYSICAL BODY CHEAT SHEET – please use this as and when is necessary, as a reference like a mini encyclopaedia.

» **Ankles** – represents the inflexibility to move forward in life. It can also be a reflection of significant control issues and a tendency to be stubborn. Also, there may be a mother conflict going on.

» **Arms** – represent an experience of powerlessness. There is usually a great fear of reclaiming your power back. If you have pain in your arm, there will likely be some changes in a relationship that is challenging right now and needs some urgent attention. Arm pain is also related to receiving and giving love since the arm leads to the heart. Left arm is receiving love, and right is giving love.

» **Bacteria** - bacterial infections like e coli represents a feeling of guilt and regret. You are great at self-punishment, you've mastered it. Consequently, this leads to self-sabotage. Your inner critic is self-violent and relentless.

» **Back** – all back issues are around some lack of support in one way or another. The back depicts the sustenance of life. Many of my clients presenting with back issues have a poor relationship with responsibility. In actuality, swinging towards taking on too much. It can be objective, but usually is mostly psychological, feeling accountable for things.

» **Breasts** – represent motherly love. Problems in this area could mean that you find it hard to give and receive nurturing love. It doesn't feel natural to you, perhaps because of your upbringing. So, you tussle with the idea of it all in your mind, and this causes a separation. Or the perception of a broken love chain.

» **Chest** – as a child, you felt pushed away by your mother. You have now mastered pushing everyone else away who is essential to you. Therefore, love has become a negative association, and you find it very difficult to express or show it. You would rather distract yourself than head this on.

- **Ears** – there is something you do not want to hear - what is that? Also, the idea of confrontation is your worst nightmare, and you feel like there could be some on the horizon if you say something, so you don't.
- **Eyes** – seeing the truth - what don't you want to see in your environment in your objective world? Is there too much responsibility in your life?
- **Fat (weight issues)** – you create a protection between you and the world by carrying excess fat, this fat represents the illusion of a barrier to protect yourself from further emotional pain. Do you feel that an influential person is a threat in your life? Have influential people not been available to you and therefore you have used food to comfort yourself?
- **Feet** – always around stepping out in the world and moving forward or being seen. It can trigger fear which in turn triggers the feeling that you're out of control. Do you feel like you've lost direction? Do you resist change? Why?
- **Heart** – you restrict yourself from receiving love. The left side represents receiving love and the right side represents giving.
- **Hips** – are you flexible in relationships? Yes or no?
- **Knees** – also correlate to moving forward in life, you are fearful of making significant changes. You tend to be influenced by the idea of what

other people may think of you, especially if you follow your own direction.

» **Lower back** – immense feelings of distress towards financial and family burdens. You feel enormous pressure, mainly the pressure you put upon yourself. You have high standards and therefore are a big self-critic. The outcome of this is that life can feel like a pressure cooker. Ready to explode at any time. The idea of continually meeting financial and family demands feels too much. You don't feel supported.

» **Middle back** - always around responsibility for others. Ask yourself if you find it hard to determine whether something is your responsibility or someone else's? This uncertainty will cast you to feel so uncomfortable that you find yourself taking it on, regardless. Sometimes you feel controlled by someone close to you in your life. Who is that? Why do you feel controlled?

» **Neck** – you find it challenging to make decisions and feel out of your depth in relationships.

Now you have had a taster of the cheat sheet above we are going to take action. You will be revisiting the metaphysical anatomy analysis while tackling the next section.

3.5.3. F.A.M. ACTION – RELEASE THE FEELINGS AND EMOTIONS AROUND YOUR PAIN

How to make THE F.A.M. METAPHYSICAL questions work for you.

» Do not think about the answers, just brainstorm whatever comes up for you.
» Do not over analyse, just trust what comes up is correct.
» Be open to answering the questions as honestly as you can, even if the answer scares you a little.
» Not all the questions will be relevant, again be open to the answer being there when it is. If there is no answer then move onto the next question.
» Take a deep breath and begin. Put pen to paper and just see what comes out.

Now time for a life changing F.A.M. exercise.

3.5.4. F.A.M. EXERCISE "FEEL, DEAL AND DUMP"

1. Take a feeling you have identified. Perhaps it is, "I feel angry at .... for calling me stupid!" Take ANGER as your title then ask yourself, "How does anger make me FEEL?" It is crucial that you focus on the emotions, the feeling and the energy and not the events around the emotion. It is the feelings that you are trying to uncover and release.

2. Keep writing until there is nothing left to come out of your pen. The writing doesn't have to be neat or grammatically correct; it is the intention which allows this process to work each time. Avoid thinking, just see what comes out of your pen - don't allow yourself to engage in thinking about the answer. Just let the flow of consciousness happen.

Ask these questions:

» What are the possible reasons for this feeling?
» What suppressed emotion am I holding on to?
» Underneath the answer, ask yourself - "what is the FEELING that I FEEL when I focus on it?"

Let me help you with a real-life example from a client who has allowed me to share this with you. A trigger for them was a previous relationship breakdown. This created a lot of suppressed, negative emotion which gave them many physical issues. Poor sleep, overthinking, worry and a lack of self-worth to name but a few. The client realised that the main feelings at the core were anger and guilt. In pinpointing the feelings from using the exercise above I asked the client to use the F.A.M. "Feel, Deal and Dump" exercise in order to move these feelings through their body. The client then spent a short 2 minutes frantically writing about those feelings relating to anger to the point where the writing became so fast and unclear it wasn't even readable. They used words and phrases such as "I can't believe how stupid I was," "frustration," "need to change." It was the third time the client had done the feel deal and dump exercise and he called me to explain how it made him feel. "I feel like I am literally having an adrenaline rush, a buzz! For the first time in years I have a knowing that everything is going to be, not just ok, but great."

A great testimonial for sure but one that also demonstrates persistence, I made the point that this was the third time the client had used the exercise, to simply show and be transparent that you must practice. "Practice makes Perfect?" I prefer; Perfect practice - makes perfect! I am sharing this with you as this exercise can seem so simple that it would be easy for you to think that it is not working, or won't work. I can assure you, there is only one rule with this type of transformation and healing and that is that you have to take action in a new way. If you do this consistently you will get the results. That I can promise. Just make sure you are working on experiencing the feelings rather than the story that accompanies them.

The primary key here is to NEVER let yourself lock onto the feeling of pain that your body is telling you, you will instantly go into resistance to the pain which will feed the pain, making it potentially worse. You have to become like a Sherlock Holmes of your thoughts, stories, unconscious behaviours and emotions. Ask yourself. What is being shown and known to you? What does this pain want you to uncover? Always ask the right questions. The mind loves to answer questions. If you don't present it with quality questions, it will make things up. By refocusing your attention to turn off resistance, you enter a state of allowing. It is the only place where true healing can happen! When we "resist, we persist!" When we "FEEL, we deal!" Simple huh!

3.5.5. F.A.M. ANTIDOTE – TRANSCEND INTO A STATE OF WELL-BEING AND ALIGNMENT

Once you have finished writing, it's time to set the paper on fire and let it burn – literally, give it back to the universe. This part is very significant as you complete a cycle of letting go. The suppressed emotion is released onto paper, and now you burn it so the cycle is complete and the suppressed emotion returns to consciousness, to God, whatever word you wish to use; it's all the same meaning. The letting go process is you letting this negative emotion free as the feeling is no longer relevant and does not serve you. It does not define you; therefore, it's time to release it.

The key point here is that you have worked through this process from within, not had to confront anyone or anything, only using your body, its feelings and this exercise to grow.

After this process, you may feel emotional; you may feel nothing, either way, is fine. There is no right or wrong way. This process is mechanical; you do it, and it works. In the case of my client I mentioned above, the first time they did the feel, deal and dump exercise, they found it interesting. They were fascinated by the idea of seeing what emotions and feelings could be hidden in their subconscious mind, the second time they said they just felt numb but the third gave them an almost euphoric feeling, like an adrenaline hit!

Now you have completed this letting go cycle it is essential you choose where your attention is going to go next. Remember where attention goes energy flows. Experience is your energy focused into an either upward or downward spiralling moments. When we feel fat, anxious, overwhelmed, low confidence etc. it is our body's compass telling us that we are out of alignment with our truth. What has happened is suppressed emotions rise, the mind then vibrationally matches that emotion with the same kind of thoughts. We grab them believing it is true as the feeling supports the thought which makes us feel rubbish. What has happened is old suppressed emotion has risen from the subconscious mind. Our job is to see all of this as an opportunity to grow. Like a gift in which we get to be grateful for. With the experience of discomfort, there has to be something we need to see, let go of and change our relationship to. A large part of this journey is not to take it seriously at all. That would also be the mind trapping you into believing that change has to be hard. In the case of my client, the gift was the pain of separation, a gift in a sense of it being a catalyst for growth!

For so long now we have been holding back, stuffing the truth (our real feelings) back into our subconscious, in fear of being judged, losing control or even worse, we were to be ostracised, and rejection became our reality. Now we get to play big and choose our focus point in life instead of drowning in regret, fear and limitation. It's time to be present and put our attention onto the expansion of now.

Ask yourself..... "who do I want to be?" (that could be a healthy version of yourself, more dynamic, confident, playful, carefree etc).

- » How does it FEEL to be this person? Write it down. Put pen to paper and let it flow. See what comes out of your pen.
- » Play with this feeling for a couple of minutes - where can you feel it in your body?
- » How intense is it out of 10 (1 = poor 10 = amazing)?

Imagine this feeling filling your entire body up like white golden liquid. Every cell of your being is vibrating with this feeling. Understand the power of the imagination and using the imagination creates abundant new neural pathways – a new place for the mind to go instead of bringing up an old habitual way of thinking.

4. CHAPTER FOUR - FREEDOM ALIGNMENT METHOD METAPHYSICAL ANATOMY

Remember not all the questions will be relevant to your situation. Be open, allow yourself to anchor in with the questions. Read one at a time, if it does resonate then record the answer.

4.1. GENERAL PHYSICAL PAIN

» Do you have any unresolved anger towards someone? If yes, who and what are the outrage and anger about?
» How does this person make you feel? (only write about how it makes you FEEL, not the story, you can use the story to get to the feeling if you need to).
» What trauma or problem were you facing when this pain began? (Listen to your gut instinct if you're not sure).
» When did your pain start?
» What stressful things were you going through at the time? Such as financial, family, work, health, overwhelm, uncertainty etc.
» Where and what are you resisting? (The more pain you are experiencing, the more resistance you have towards expressing yourself).
» Do you feel you deserve the punishment of pain?
» Do you find it hard to say no? What stops you?
» What do you feel guilty about in life?

- Is there a situation or a person in your life that was making you feel trapped when the pain began (and potentially currently too)?
- What have you been doing against your will? (be honest).
- Do you find yourself focused on the issues that currently bother you? Perhaps, you notice you talk about or think about a negative problem, for example, an external one such as blame (it is someone else's fault) rather than looking at what is going on for you? What was going on for you emotionally, when the pain began?
- Does your pain flare up when you're around certain people or particular environments? Be observant - look at what is going on in your life when the pain gets worse. I have had many clients who, when heading home after a weekend away or to the office on a Monday morning find the pain increases tenfold. The environment can be a massive trigger for stress.
- Sometimes the anxiety/stress is going on in your mind. The trigger happens when you are focused on a negative story - often in a future moment. For example, you are worried about a meeting at work, an awkward conversation you must have. A truth you must share, an ending of some partnership, romantic or business.

TIP: The story you tell yourself about who you think you are or are not, if negative, will keep you trapped. Become aware of what you are telling yourself and others. Listen to the language you use to others to describe who you are. Does your story need re-writing? If there is any hint of being the victim in your story, then you are in a trap! YOU MUST re-write your story to free yourself from the trap. Why? You have learnt that it doesn't serve you to blame the outside – it serves you to deal with your own inner world. Being a victim will keep you stuck in the belief that there is nothing YOU can do to change or get better. But all you need to do is release the emotion. Victim (it's not fair) or blame is of a vibration that matches resistance. Resistance keeps you in the same repetitive behaviours and thinking as before. You already know what you have been doing doesn't work. So as Einstein so wonderfully said: "We can't solve problems by using the same kind of thinking we used when we created them." The healing process is no different; you have to behave and think in a different way to be freed from that which keeps you stuck; victim stories are subtle traps.

4.2. SHOULDER PAIN

Do you feel like you are carrying the weight of the world on your shoulders? Pain in the shoulders is always a sign of some considerable amount of perceived and actual responsibilities. Be honest, make a list of all the responsibilities you have going on in all areas of your life now. Go to the following topics below and write out for each one what responsibilities you have.

Look at:

- Work
- Home
- Relationships
- Finances
- Self-development
- Family/children
- Health

Now, answer the following questions. Do not overthink the answers. Just ask yourself the question and see what comes out of your pen. Not all the questions will be relevant so focus on the ones that have resonance.

- Do you feel weighed down with responsibility? If so, why?
- Are you still willing to take on more responsibility even though you are bogged down with things to do? If so, why?
- Do you measure your value by how much you do for others?

- Is there a sense that you can't stop taking more on? Is it because you have a strong sense of not wanting to let anyone down?
- Does the thought of letting someone down fill you with dread and guilt?
- Do you have low self-esteem?
- Does your low self-esteem often sabotage your ability to express clear boundaries?
- Do you find it hard to trust others to be able to do the job as well as you?
- Do you find yourself supporting others because it makes you feel valued? Or is it through guilt, fear or habit?
- Do you notice you like to try and control outcomes in life?
- Are you controlling?
- Does this make you feel safe?
- Do you crave acceptance and praise? How does that make you feel?
- Do you feel that people want too much from you? If so, why?
- Do you feel angry and resentful?
- Do you feel that you get taken advantage of by friends and work colleagues?

4.3. LEFT SHOULDER

» Do you have financial responsibilities that feel overwhelming?
» Do you feel responsible for co-workers and or a partner?
» The left side is the feminine side - what female in your life is putting responsibilities on your shoulders? Mother, friend, sister, daughter, work colleague? How does that make you feel?
» Have you made a decision that made you feel disempowered? If so, what and why?

4.4. RIGHT SHOULDER

» Do you feel that you have lots of family responsibilities.
» Do you think that you have lots of work responsibilities?
» This is the masculine side - is there a male in your life, currently, who appears to be putting more responsibilities onto your shoulders?
» Are you responsible for pleasing your father?
» Do you have any male in your life who is putting lots of responsibility on you?

4.5. SHOULDER BLADES

- Is there a female in your life who is challenging your confidence and determination to be successful? If so, who and how does that make you feel?
- Do you feel controlled or under attack?
- Do you feel attacked by a feminine figure in your life?
- Do you feel humiliated and intimidated by someone in the family or close to you?
- Do you feel powerless?
- If so, why? Describe the feeling of "powerlessness."
- Do you feel unsupported? If so, why do you and what other feelings do you associate with being "unsupported?"

4.6. FEET

We use the feet to physically move forward and metaphysically they also represent our ability to emotionally move forward in life. The foot is always significant to this. Now ask yourself the following:

- Do you fear standing up for yourself?
- Do you have a fear of your future?
- Do you fear losing control?
- Do you fear moving forward in life?
- Do you fear potential success?

- Have you had a shortage of support and guidance in the past?
- When going through something new in your life, have you struggled with support?
- What lousy experience have you had, especially around a change of direction in life?
- Have you been criticised for this, if so when, who and why? How did it make you feel?
- Have you been punished or abused by an influential and controlling person when you made changes?
- Do you fear change?
- What is it about change that scares you?
- Do you fear commitment?
- Have you suppressed your ability to make decisions in fear of influential people telling you you're wrong or incapable?
- Do you doubt your ability to be successful and therefore don't make changes quickly? Stay stuck in your current place - yet feel unfulfilled or unhappy?
- Do you believe making change is dangerous, who in your life had this fear?
- Do you feel stubborn, rigid and inflexible in regards to change? If so, which one more?
- What would happen if you were to physically and or mentally become still and stop? How does it make you feel?
- When did the foot problem begin?

- What was happening in your life during this time?
- What stress around change and moving forward was going on?

4.7. ANKLES

Swollen ankles reflect resentment and 'being stuck' in your life. It can be a drama in your life which you feel there is no solution or immediate light at the end of the tunnel. It can be an inner frustration. Sometimes you may feel like you are getting yourself into a pickle. Especially if your intentions were pure and supportive and yet your experience is the opposite of this. Answer the questions below, remember not all of them will be relevant so don't think, just focus on the ones that feel true. Then ask yourself, how does the answer to the question make you "feel?" Write it out.

- Who or what do you resent, especially around the time the ankle started to swell?
- Is there any alcohol abuse in your life? If so, who is the abuser and how does this make you feel?
- Are you stubborn? How does the stubbornness serve you?
- What would happen if you let go of the stubbornness?
- How would that make you feel?
- Do you have any frustration and trauma related to being controlled by a feminine figure?

- » If yes, how does that make you feel?
- » Do you have a fear of standing your ground?
- » What would happen if you did stand your ground? How does that make you feel?
- » Do you feel unworthy or not allowed to stand your ground?

4.8. BACK PAIN

The back is always a representation of a lack of support. The back supports the entire body. Therefore, it is the first place to show pain when you have a conscious or unconscious belief, idea, story that you are not supported.

The Coccyx/Sacrum (base of the spine) this pain represents self-pity. You find it excruciating to ask for help, so instead, you wallow in self-pity. Problems in this area happen when we refuse to reach out, feel ashamed to ask for help and will cut our noses off to spite our face. We then feel internally sad that people are not running to our rescue.

- » Do you fear you will lose your freedom by being in pain?
- » Is your freedom compromised?
- » Do you ever fear getting better?
- » Do you overthink and worry about the worst-case outcome?

- Do others need your help which you feel is threatening to you, as this equals less time which is less freedom?
- Are you frustrated?

I experienced this. One day, I felt my back "go," Why? Because I was fuming with my sons and forgot to let them into the internal battle I had going on. Instead, I internally fought until the next day when I woke up, I couldn't move. I felt as though they were not supportive of me because I had 3 strapping teenagers that just left me to get on with moving my office, on my own, not taking any initiative to help me. I did laugh as I found myself doing the "Feel, deal and dump" exercise. The results? Anger, resentment, frustration, total disappointment. The problem was that I had held on to the thoughts and thinking of resentment, "the boys have let me down" etc. to the point where one negative thought lead to another. My awareness of this allowed me my biggest learning. That of the need to surrender. Once I had let go, through the Feel, Deal & Dump process, within 24 hours, I could move with ease again. No doubt if I had not used the process, I would have been out of sorts for at least a week or more.

4.9. LOWER BACK PAIN

- » Do you feel unsupported? Period!
- » Do you worry about money?
- » Do you worry about the family?
- » Do you feel that you have to do everything yourself?
- » Do you feel that others may not be there for you?
- » Do you find it hard to receive?
- » Do you find it hard to give?
- » Can you allow yourself to accept things?
- » Do you feel secure in your life?
- » Do you fear losing material possessions?
- » Do you also recognise that you don't want to admit this to yourself?

4.10. UPPER BACK PAIN

- » Does having back pain give you a secondary gain like not having to do everything for everyone else? Sometimes do you just want a break from it all?
- » Do you expect a lot from others, and if they do not meet your expectations you can feel let down?
- » Do you feel like you have a lot on your back?
- » Do you feel stuck?

- Do you feel that you need to make sure everyone is happy all the time?
- Are you terrible at asking for help?
- Do you feel you lack emotional security?
- Do you feel that you need to be continually doing things?
- If someone does something for you, do you feel loved and secure?
- Is your way of showing love through doing things?

4.11. SCIATIC PAIN

Your sciatic nerve is the main nerve that runs down your leg. All nerve pain is related to communication and sensitivity. You are not saying what's really on your mind.

- Do you feel that you need more support?
- Do you feel that you can't cope with everything on your own?
- Do you feel you cannot stand up for yourself?
- Are you not communicating properly?
- Is there a situation that you cannot take any longer? If so, what is it and why can't you stand it anymore? How does it make you feel?
- Do you fear where you are going in your life?
- Do you feel that you won't be able to cope with what lies ahead?

» Do you feel that something or someone is restricting your freedom?
» Do you feel financial burdens?
» Do you feel emotional burdens?

4.12. NECK PAIN

The neck moves gracefully from left to right allowing you to have flexibility. When there is a pain in the neck, then you have left creativity and entered into fear and have repressed self-expression along the way. It can mean there is someone who is being a "pain in the neck" in your life right now. Who is that? Why are they and how does it make you feel?

» Who is being a pain in your neck in your life right now? (a person or people)
» Do you need to be in control?
» Are you uncomfortable expressing your dislikes in life?
» Are you analytical and avoid feelings at all costs?
» Do you have trust issues?

4.13. HEADACHES

Head pain always indicates separation and resistance to what is in your objective world. There is a separation from your truth. The greater the pain, the more important that something is. Perhaps fear of messing things up. Each part of the head represents a different emotional trigger. The top of the head (Vertex) area is associated with our connection to the Universe or God. If you have pain here, it means you are experiencing a disconnection from that higher power. In Chinese medicine, it is linked with the Kidneys which are connected to fear. The forehead area is connected to your 3rd eye. Pain here is associated with the "illusion of separation" from yourself. Self-love and the need to have an inward practice such as meditation is paramount to shifting your relationship to pain here.

Occipital area; The back of the head represents your past. Pain here represents something in your past that is not complete and remains unforgiven. Anger and resentment builds from the reluctance of fear of heading this on and dealing with it. Pain in the back of the head represents a total unwillingness to dive deep inwards. It happens when you're spending too much time in your head thinking, obsessing analysing, rationalising, speculating, worrying, organising or feeling lost.

Temporal; The sides of the head are associated with courage, especially courage to face your world. Migraine headaches, usually located in the front quadrants, right or left, indicates an illusion of separation from your world, from your objective world.

The involvement of the eyes in migraines indicate not only an unwillingness to look outwards but to look within as well. Lack of joy (with one's self is the best way to sum this up). The more pain, then the less joy is happening in your experience right now. Often those who suffer from pain here really need to stop taking everything so seriously. Spend time looking at the meaning you have been attributing to things, people and events in your life. Does it need a serious update? Then go and answer the following questions. Again, do not overthink this, just see what comes out of your pen. Then go back and read what you have put.

- What are you resisting in your life right now?
- Who are you resisting?
- Do you feel frustrated, if so, what or who with?
- Do you feel rigid in your life, almost stuck?
- Is there something or someone you are avoiding?
- Is there an imbalance going on? Too much focus on mind, not enough on heart?
- Are you trying too hard?
- Do you feel angry?

4.14. MIGRAINES

Migraines occur because of imploding emotions such as irritation and anger. Migraines appear when you are in resistance to something in your world. If I have ever started with a migraine, I can usually switch them off if

I STOP (which is one of the things a migraine is trying to get you to do, because what you are doing, focusing on, thinking about, obsessing about is not serving you). I close my eyes and rest into the feeling, take the label off and just relax. This takes you out of trying to resist or control the experience into allowing it which will then shift the experience. However, if you are prone to lots of migraines, then try the questions below.

» Do you have a fear of failure?
» Do you have high expectations of yourself?
» Do you have a fear of not being able to meet these expectations?
» Did this expectation come from your parents?
» Do you have control issues?
» Do you feel trapped?
» Are you unable to take the pressure?

4.15. ANXIETY

Anxiety is the sense that something out there, in the future, seems scary. The good news is that anxiety rises to push you to deal with unresolved trauma from the past. In other words, suppressed emotions that are stuck in your subconscious and want to go. It is a good thing as it shows you that you are ready to let go of this now. It's always future worries!

The other thing to highlight is that no one has ever died of anxiety. Even though, when you are in an acute state of anxiety, you may feel like you are. The mind is running away with itself, fantasising about the worst-case scenarios. Answer the following questions.

» Are you consciously aware that you are always lost in thought and or worry?
» Do you worry a lot? If so, what about?
» Do you have a fear of urgency?
» Do you have a feeling of panic?
» Does your mind race?
» Do you worry about everyday things? (Such as work? Finances? Family?)
» Can you switch off?
» How are you in a social gathering?
» How do you feel about being the centre of attention?
» Do you fear being alone? If so, why and how does it make you feel?
» Do you have a fear of failure?
» Do you feel like a failure?
» Do you feel helpless?
» Do you feel shameful?
» Was your sense of peace regularly interrupted as a child?
» How did that make you feel?
» As a child, did you have emotional structure and or stability?

- Have you got emotional structure and or stability as an adult?
- Do you notice that your thoughts are future thoughts?
- How often do you think about the future? Daily, hourly, minute to minute?
- Are your thoughts obsessive?
- Do you currently feel trapped in your circumstances?
- Do you lack the freedom to make daily choices?
- Do you catch yourself behaving in ways to please others in fear of being judged, abused or punished?
- Does it feel safer to be someone else rather than being yourself? Does this protect you from criticism?
- Can you mis-interpret how others are communicating to you?
- Do you read into what people say too much?
- Do you fear taking on responsibility?
- Is overwhelm an issue?
- As a child, do/did you feel that there is no one to defend, protect or love you?
- Do you feel emotionally needy and insecure?
- How does anxiety serve you?
- Does it keep you safe?
- Have you made changes in your life that have resulted in a negative outcome?
- Do you fear the worst outcome?

» Do you feel needy?
» Do you believe this could lead back to being criticised or rejected?
» What is this the main thing you're trying to avoid?

4.16. PANIC ATTACKS

It is a real physiological experience in most cases; you are not going mad. During a panic attack, adrenaline and cortisol release from the brain and flood into the body, which is fine if you are running for your life. However, if sat watching T.V. perhaps at a social function or just in your office, the surge of energy these hormones create can feel like you are dying. It's almost like an internal tap gets left on, the hormones are in full flow, with nowhere to go. They start to flood your system.

Anxiety can seem like it comes out of nowhere. A real physical and mental experience, as I heard Dr Joe Dispenza say; "the body becomes the mind." The reason it happens is the mind becomes practised in catastrophising about a future moment. What if this goes wrong, what if that goes wrong. This instantly puts the body into survival mode or 'fight or flight'. After many years of practice, the body will now trigger itself into survival automatically. A massive trigger for this is over-analysing. I have many male clients who are analysts by nature, and in business, this serves them very well. However, they forget to switch it off, and it becomes an obsession. I say male because they can be (not in all cases) prominently more left brain and this is where the analytical mind lives.

Sometimes the thoughts are based on past experiences which we then catapult into the future. By grabbing hold of those thoughts and replaying them in our minds, it keeps the cortisol flowing. The alarm bell is triggered, now the mind thinks you are under attack: a severe threat is upon you. It has listened to the identification of the narrative, not knowing that this is just a future imaginary thought.

The body again becomes flooded with hormones, adrenaline and cortisol, and here we go again, you start to experience physical symptoms like increased blood pressure, heart rate etc. What also happens is your thoughts begin to match the vibration of the intense emotion, creating many more negative thoughts, which also feel real. The worst thing you can do is identify with the thought, which is what most people do. It creates more resistance which in turn creates more negative thought and more cortisol in the body. The result of all of this is a panic attack or a bad episode of anxiety.

"We have zero control over the past and zero control of the future - we only have now!"

How to STOP the panic attack.

To stop it, we need to do the opposite of what we have been doing. We must go from fighting it to allowing it.

To allow it:

» As soon as you notice you are starting to feel anxious and it's turning into a panic attack.

» STOP

» Take three HUGE breathes in - hold for five seconds on each inhale. Then exhale and push out as much air as you can. It is vital to get the oxygen back into the brain and body. Often when we start with a panic attack, our breathing gets very shallow, and this adds to the feeling of light-headedness.

» Now, take the label off the experience. For example: "oh no, I am having a panic attack, I feel like I am dying."

» This next part is crucial. Now go to the feeling behind the dialogue (this could be an anxiety feeling). Now feel the sensation underneath the label - melt into it.

» Every time your mind takes you off into thought and story again, come back and tell yourself you are feeling this feeling with every cell of your body. It will take 68 seconds to start to dissipate. You can say in your head. "I'm going to feel this with every cell of my body" over and over again if need be.

- » Now, get up and move your body. Make a cup of herbal tea, stretch, go outside, anything to move the body.
- » Finally, use an affirmation such as "I am healthy" "I am calm." Put your attention now onto something upward spiralling. Where attention goes energy flows. It is essential to choose where you put your attention next - consciously.

If it doesn't disappear the first time, that's fine, just do it again. It may come back, slightly less intense. That's fine too, just keep repeating the above exercise. It will eventually go. It is important that you break the cycle with the affirmation. You do not have to believe the words but you need a new focal point for your thoughts.

The subconscious mind has only one job to do, and that is to follow instruction from the conscious mind. Most people's subconscious minds are left to run wild and continuously think worrying self-sabotaging thoughts. If you are to continually identify with a negative narrative such as "I am stupid" "I am not liked," your objective world will start to mirror this. Where attention goes energy flows. It also works on the flip side - positive direction/ affirmations like "I am amazing" will even begin to mirror in your objective world. We attract what we focus on.

It takes 21 days to reprogram the mind. For the next 21 days set yourself a challenge to do this exercise every day. Firstly, every morning focus yourself for 90 seconds, perhaps even while brushing your teeth. Take one thing you are grateful for. Then tell yourself the reason "why" you are thankful for this thing or person. Alternatively, start the day with a power statement about yourself. A positive statement about you that begins with "I am..." Then follow the start of this statement with some positive words, for example. "I am amazing, kind, helpful, fun.....etc." You don't have to believe this statement as the subconscious mind has no idea what is real or not. This exercise will start to shift your state very quickly. Where attention goes, energy flows, remember. This exercise will shift your focus - gratitude automatically turns into a state of love. You focus long enough on this; it changes every cell in your body.

4.17. DEPRESSION

Depression or low mood. This experience, when in it, can feel like you will never be able to get out of it. It can suck you into negative dialogue, so much so it seemingly feels like there is no way out. It's NOT true, however, that's not what you want to hear when you are in it! Nor should you say that to someone who is in a low mood. Instead, it is about understanding how to move out of the experience. Believe it or not, not even a manic depressive can be depressed all the time. It takes effort. Usually something goes wrong in the person's world - an expectation is not met. The mind has an idea of life needing to look a certain way. When the hope doesn't match the person's ideas, it is easy to grab onto the negative dialogue. The dialogue sounds something like: "but why" "it's not fair" "bad things always happen to me." This can spiral someone into a pool of intense emotions which feel cumbersome, demotivating and make you feel powerless. How do you snap out of it? You head on the reasons/feelings why you are feeling this in the first place. You STOP resisting the experience, and you start to allow it by "feeling the feeling." Let's find out where you are at.

» Do you feel devalued? - if so, why and how does it make you feel?
» What passion do you disconnect yourself from in life?
» What is your life purpose? Do you know?
» What excites you in life?
» What are you good at?
» Do you feel misunderstood by people?
» If so, by whom and how does that make you feel?
» Do you feel that you need to give up because there are no options?
» Do you feel you have lost your sense of hope?
» Are you judgemental?
» Do you try and hide how you feel because you don't want others to judge you?

- » When did the depression start?
- » What was happening in your life when the depression started?
- » What is your relationship with your parents like?
- » Is there an unresolved issue?
- » What secondary gains does the depression give you?
- » Does this condition make it easier for you to express your boundaries?
- » Do you feel safer when you're feeling like this?
- » Has depression become your label?
- » Are there responsibilities in your life that may make you feel overwhelmed?
- » Who do you see yourself as?
- » How does leaving your comfort zone make you feel?
- » Do you feel a lot of shame?
- » Do you feel guilty?
- » Do you feel that you have to hide how are you feeling from others?
- » Do you feel that you only get noticed when you behave in a certain way?

Now you have established your metaphysical connection, it is time to work through the root causes of your pain and let go of the suppressed emotions attached to the particular block or problem. It is also important to highlight at this point that if you are struggling to work through your own emotional, mental and or physical pain then please do not panic. Sometimes you need an external perspective from someone impartial. I am sure we have all experienced seeing something in someone that the individual is unaware of.

5. CHAPTER FIVE - FREEDOM ALIGNMENT METHOD

5.1. FEEL DEAL AND DUMP CONTINUED

When we feel we deal - this process is how we transcend pain and suffering. Most of our lives we have been pushing or stuffing our feelings away. The unlearning of such behaviours is the only challenge you will have, purely because the programme to "push" or "stuff" the emotion will be so ingrained that you will be doing this unconsciously. Do not worry. If there is pain, then you already have enough emotion floating to the surface to "feel, deal & dump." If you are currently pain free it means your subconscious doesn't feel that there is any need for you to let go of the repressed emotions at this moment. So, enjoy!

Ask yourself the following questions. The first question is probably one of the most essential questions you could ask yourself from this book. It will give you some real insight into what stress is mirroring the suppressed emotions and therefore has a need to be removed.

- When did the pain start?
- If the pain could speak to you, what would it say?
- What does it need?
- How can I live a life where the pain is NO LONGER necessary?

The fastest way to "feel and deal" is to make life a playful game of letting go! Which of course, HAS to be a conscious choice. Are you ready to let go of the physical, mental or emotional pain?

» What do I need to let go of?
» Ask the body parts that are in pain; what do I need to see, hear, feel and or let go of?
» What negative emotion do I need to feel and deal with?

Now see what comes out of your pen. Journaling can take a few minutes before the stream of consciousness, and answers start to appear, try to be patient. By the way, not everyone is a natural at this so, like I say, be patient with yourself. You may find it difficult mainly because your mind is trying to overthink the process. The best tip I can give you is to TRUST - whatever comes out of your pen, even if it doesn't make sense, it is right.

The next important part of this exercise is to use the answers to your best advantage. For example: "I feel angry at my partner, friend, parent etc." Take this answer, pop it at the top of an empty page and ask yourself, "how does this honestly make me FEEL." Let your pen flow, if you notice your mind is getting involved then you're trying to think about the answers. Stop. Take a deep breath then dive back into the question again. This time allowing the answers to stream out of your pen. Do not stop until there is nothing left to write. It is vital that you write about the feelings and not the story. As feeling the feeling will put you into a state of "allowing." Talking about the story will put you into a state of resistance. Healing happens when we allow.

Do this exercise for everything that came up in your answers. You can do this exercise as many times as you need to. In the beginning you will find there is more letting go to do so please do not worry if you find yourself doing this exercise a few times a day. The more pain the more letting go is needed. The exercise is life changing and powerful. However, you may have a life time of suppressed emotions to allow and let go of. So be patient and please do not give up after the first go. This is a journey not a destination and the more unattached to the outcome you become the quicker the results will be.

As this is an extension of the Feel, Deal and Dump exercise from earlier remember to do the same when you have written out what has come up for you, so, take the paper and burn it! Letting go, an energetic release. Giving the energy back to where it belongs- back to consciousness, back to the universe!

An additional example of the "Feel, Deal and Dump" Freedom Alignment Method Exercise:

A client had really bad anxiety and shoulder pain. She arrived saying she had tried everything. Nothing was working and now her problems were starting to affect all areas of her life. The physical pain in her shoulder was stopping her driving, playing with her children and was terribly embarrassing at work when she was struggling to lift things.

Emotionally, the anxiety was stopping her taking action with new and exciting work events and socially, she started to turn into a recluse.

On arriving to the sessions, I asked her if she was stressed? She said no more than any other working mum. I asked her if she had had anxiety for a long time. She said it was something she recognised being there, on and off in her life for many years but was now affecting her sleep and making her feel unworthy. She also felt that as a consequence, she had put on a lot of weight which was compounding the way she saw herself and how she thought others saw her too.

So, I asked her two simple questions.

- When did the anxiety and shoulder pain start?
- What stressful things were going on in her life at the time?

I received the answers, albeit after doing some digging. It is not always surface stress that triggers these things, it can be triggered through worrying about things, obsessing over something or just overthinking worst case scenarios which haven't even happened yet.

It was clear she felt that all the responsibilities were on her shoulders, the children, family, out of school clubs she was running, work commitments, finances etc and she was feeling unconsciously resentful about this. She hadn't realised that she had not said "no" for years. Admittedly, partly because she felt immense guilt which drove her to always say "yes" when she really meant "NO."

So, we took the title "I feel resentful for all the responsibility I have." She then did the "feel, deal and dump" exercise using this title. Lots of emotions like anger, rage, irritation and guilt came flowing out, which was fantastic.

This started to ease the pain in her shoulders. The next move was to then take action on saying "NO." Today she has mastered the ability to say "no" with zero guilt. Her pain has gone and she feels amazing. She also did the "feel, deal and dump" with her anxiety which has also disappeared too. This has now triggered her to lose weight too.

The main reason her results are so fantastic is because she kept on doing the "feel, deal and dump," when needed.

5.2. ANTIDOTE – THE F.A.M. UPWARD SPIRALLING CREATOR EXERCISE

Before we jump into this method, I want to make it clear what this isn't. It is NOT an opportunity to think positively. Under no circumstances am I promoting thinking!! All thinking is a trap, positive or not! It will always lead you onto some downward spiralling negative thinking lane which will encourage a focus on what you don't want. It is what most people are unconsciously addicted to.

You may use a word or a thought to get to the vibration of what you want but you must then put the thought down. Do NOT entertain a story or thinking process. Studies have shown that if you think about something long enough, it will always become negative. It is the nature of the egoic mind. Remember the ego will always look for problems.

This exercise is about creating an intention and then letting go of that intention, swapping it for the vibration the intention gives you.

To be honest, the magic takes just 20 seconds to start working. Note that after one minute you will be strengthening a strong vibration of desire, you will be unknowingly portraying this out to the universe. This is basic physics. We live in a vibrational universe. The universal language is energy/vibration. In order to create something, you have to become the vibrational match to that which you desire. So become joy, become love and peace and see how easy life gets. The more familiar you make this feeling, the quicker the results. A great line sung by Paula Abdul says; "you give love, you get love."

Ask yourself the following questions and be honest.
What is it that this new way of being will bring me?

So, for example, if it's more money, what is it more money brings you? For me, it is always about having the freedom to do what I want, when I want. Yours may be love, a new job, more money, health, better relationships etc.

Finally, you now know what the new way of being is. The next step is for you to find the feeling of this new way of being. You must spend time mastering this as this is when shifting and creating begins. You have got to experience the ultimate upward spiralling feeling in this moment, right now and start building this into your reality.

How does joy, freedom and or peace feel like to you? Where in your physical body do you feel that?

The more familiar you are at resting into this experience, the more you become this and therefore become a matching vibration to that with which you wish to attract. Where attention goes energy flows, as mentioned many times before. All matter, including thoughts, emotions etc. can be broken down into vibrational energy resonating at different levels, we live in a vibrational universe.

All you need to do is now rest into that feeling with every cell of your body, this is a crucial part - as you shift your vibration into a new upward spiralling state - it's like having a love affair with the very feeling you desire to have.

Once you have started to feel it in your experience it is time to ask yourself "where in my body do I feel this again?"

Once you have identified this, mark the intensity out of 10, how strongly do you feel this in your body?

Now, turn it up to a 7 in intensity in your body. Feel it, really FEEL it and then turn it up to a 10....... imagine it's like a huge volume dial on your chest, now allow yourself to feel this in every cell of your body. Can you do it? Can you feel it now?

Don't stop untill you can!

You should have an embodied experience of that feeling. Sometimes the mind will kick in and try to divert you away from the feeling. That's ok, gently bring yourself back to the upward spiralling feeling you are desiring.

Your homework over the next 24 hours is to make this experience the most significant love affair you have ever experienced. Play big and see how fun you can make this. Perhaps have some reminders such as brushing your teeth, driving the car, taking the dog for a walk. Every time, remembering to rest into the feeling.

When I ask people what they want out of life. They sometimes say materialistic things like money, new house etc, but mostly they are desiring the feeling these things give them. I can guarantee that if someone says money and I then ask them, "what will money give you?" In all cases, it is happiness, contentment, freedom etc. The responses always come back to a way that they want to feel. Mostly we all want to feel fulfilled, happy, loved, connected, at peace etc. Everything we do is because we are after a feeling. The money may seem like the driving force but the reality is that the cash brings you freedom, choice, peace and the ability to make a difference to other people's lives, people who you love and care for. The truth is, it's not the money you're after its the feeling the money provides you. So how exciting is it that you can create the very emotion you so desire by tapping into that feeling, focusing on it even before you have the actual thing you wished for. Magic.

The next focus point is to harness this experience by doing it every day and every time you notice your mind wandering off, trying to work problems out - STOP, give no more attention to ANY issues. Stop yourself from complaining and only focus on what you want. Mostly you will notice your mind is very good at focusing on what you don't want. This is a trap and will keep you stuck in a loop. Shift your focus, no matter what is going on in your life. Stop and transfer your attention to a higher vibrational feeling. One that you desire.

Where attention goes energy flows remember! It is why the only thing ever to protest is PEACE! You can't fight for peace only give peace for peace!

Now keep repeating and watch your life transform! BOOM!

Basic rules of embodying your highest vibrational experience.

- Always feel your way into this state; don't do what most people do. Don't keep your focus on downward spiralling emotions. You only have to go down to your local supermarket and overhear people's conversations. Often, there is lots of moaning about life's problems and dramas. Discussions on what they haven't got and how they don't like this, and don't like that. It is incredible how cornered these conversations keep people.
- If that is you then the best way to move through the negative dialogue is to, "Feel deal and dump" them, whenever they present themselves to you. Then, be a conscious creator and put your attention on the FEELING of that which you desire. Play with the universal language of energy, awe and play BIG. Remember, like attracts like, magnets are drawn to each other, allow yourself to feel your way to your dream life. To get love, you give love, dream big.
- Become it - simply become the feeling.
- Your inner being is all over it, it knows it and will support it once you match it.
- The new empowering information will stratospherically transform you into a productive application of creating - consistently and

consciously. Being a creator ensures continual growth.

» When you are in a place of stillness, there is no thought; this is where opportunity unfolds.
» An impulse or intuitive thought will now present itself, see it and follow it. Never underestimate your intuition.
» When you are in this state of stillness - you have access to what your inner being knows. Now follow your being and discover your real power.
» Feel what you want! FEEL, FEEL, FEEL!

Once you have done this the final step is........

Ask yourself:

» What do I want to have more of in my life?
» Is it an abundance of connection with my children, more constant income, love, commitment, fun, joy, laughter, support, exercise, health, opportunities, open minded people, spiritual opportunity? From resistance to allowing, a formula you should spend time mastering.

For more in depth help with this, it is perhaps necessary for you to work with someone to metaphorically hold your hand through the process. Someone who, is not only unattached emotionally to both your life and circumstances but has a passion to work with and help heal humanity. A person with an abundance of training in human behaviour, coaching, metaphysics, meditation and over a decade of experience in working with thousands of other clients around the globe; you will get highly desired results - fast. If this is you then please go to the back of the book where you can find out how you can get in touch.

5.3. CORE VALUES EXERCISE

Like all exercises in this book, must be done from a present expansive space. Look at the list below of values and circle the ones that resonate with you. Of course, if there is a word that isn't on there then pop it down.

» Accepting
» Able
» Amenable
» Alert
» Accountable
» Adaptable
» Ambitious
» Attentive
» Abundant
» Achiever
» Awareness
» Assertive
» Bold
» Brave
» Brilliant
» Balanced
» Beautiful
» Calm
» Capable
» Certainty
» Cheeky
» Clear
» Comfortable
» Communication
» Competence
» Connection
» Contribution
» Committed
» Consistent
» Conviction
» Creativity
» Courage
» Curious
» Careful
» Clever
» Common sense
» Compassion
» Confident
» Contentment
» Credible
» Dedicated
» Driven

» Divine
» Determined
» Decisive
» Disciplined
» Dynamic
» Effective
» Empowered
» Expressive
» Energetic
» Enthusiastic
» Excellent
» Empathetic
» Free
» Fun
» Fearless
» Focused
» Fair
» Foresightful
» Genuine
» Giving
» Grateful
» Greatness
» Growth
» Good
» Generous
» Hilarious
» Happy
» Honest
» Hopeful
» Humorous
» Healthy
» Intelligent
» Intuitive
» Imaginative
» Independent
» Innovative
» Inquisitive
» Individual
» Insightful
» Inspirational
» Integral
» Kind
» Knowledgeable
» Liberal
» Logical
» Loving
» Loyal
» Meaningful
» Moderate
» Motivational
» Open
» Optimistic
» Organised
» Passionate
» Patient
» Peaceful
» Persistent
» Professional
» Prosperity
» Purposeful
» Playful
» Powerful
» Present
» Productive
» Respectful
» Responsible
» Realistic
» Reflective
» Significance
» Silence
» Simplicity
» Safe
» Sexy
» Skilful
» Smart
» Spiritual
» Spontaneous
» Support
» Selfless
» Sensitive
» Strong
» Success
» Sustainable
» Thorough
» Thoughtful
» Tolerance
» Traditional

- » Talented
- » Thankful
- » Transparent
- » Trustworthy
- » Trusting
- » Tranquil
- » Understanding
- » Unique
- » Visionary
- » Wealthy
- » Welcoming
- » Wise

Take the words that you have circled and mark them out of 10 of importance, 1 having no resonance and 10 being integral to your being. If you are unsure about what is important to you, think of a time when you were most content and happy, these times are almost always because you are in alignment with your core values. Just ask yourself the question "How important is this?" And whatever number comes up in your awareness, assign the word that number.

Now take the six words that scored the highest for you and ask yourself:

- » How does the 'word' make me feel?
- » Does the 'word' feel consistent with who I am?
- » Is there a gap or am I living the life aligned with my value?

When to use your core values in your life to your advantage:

When making a decision, you must ask yourself if it is in alignment with your core values. Be honest with yourself - when I am doing something that is not aligned with my truth, my values, I always get a feeling in the pit of my stomach, like an inner signal. I haven't always listened to that feeling or sign however, the more aware of these things I became, the easier it was to notice the inner compass.

- Do you spend your time generally in alignment with your core values?
- Are you inspired by how you invest your time? Be it reading a book or going for a walk?
- What lights you up?
- Knowingness?

By checking in with yourself and asking these questions, you will ensure that you are always in alignment. It is more important than you may realise. My spiritual teacher Maharishi Krisnanda Ishaya once said to me, when I asked him if doing a new training programme served me, "does it excite you? If it does, then go for it." Excitement is a sign you're on the right track-in alignment with your inner knowing, your truth.

6. CHAPTER SIX - I WANT TO KNOW MORE. WHAT CAN I DO?

If you feel like you would like some extra help on returning yourself to empowerment and health, then book a FREE Discovery Session with the Freedom Alignment Team.

6.1. DISCOVERY SESSION

» 1-2-1 over Zoom, WhatsApp or face to face.
» Introduction to the Freedom Alignment Method, what the process is and how it addresses physical, emotional and mental pain.
» A chance for you to ask questions.
» A mini health assessment so that we can identify what possibilities there are for you going forward.
» Finally, based on the results, share with you, a bespoke programme option that will serve you the most.
» The session is approx. 45 minutes long.
» Contact us: *www.kirsty-bortoft.com* or *hello@kirsty-bortoft.com*

Go to the link to meet Kirsty
in a short free masterclass

https://go.kirsty-bortoft.com/call-s

6.2. THE BRIGHT PATH ASCENSION MEDITATION

What is Ascension?

"The Bright Path Ishayas. Ascension is for anyone seeking inner peace, happiness, freedom from stress, and a living experience of love, presence and oneness. "Ishaya" is a Sanskrit word that means, "for higher consciousness." The Ishayas are devoted to experiencing and helping others experience higher states of human consciousness. Most of us only know ourselves as a bundle of thoughts, beliefs, opinions and judgments. These are the source of all of our stress, limitations, problems and suffering. Beyond the constant chatter of the surface of the mind, is an endless well-spring of peace, joy, creativity and freedom. Ascension is a tool to help you access these extraordinary states as a direct, living experience. This teaching offers a scarce opportunity to experience what it means to be truly alive."

For First Sphere meditation course dates and times go to the following website:

https://www.thebrightpath.com

6.3. HOW TO CONTACT THE F.A.M. TEAM

LinkedIn	*https://bit.ly/2HSGYeQ*
Facebook	*https://bit.ly/3mHZrd4*
Instagram	*https://bit.ly/2HThRs2*
Website	*www.kirsty-bortoft.com*
Email	*hello@kirsty-bortoft.com*

6.4. ABOUT THE AUTHOR

Fifteen years ago, I felt pain daily. I had horrible anxiety and began experiencing panic attacks out of the blue. Often, I thought I was dying; the mental pain in my head was relentless. It was an inner self-critic which wouldn't go away!

Life seemed like it couldn't get any worse, but I was wrong; it did. I found myself homeless, penniless, scared and to top it off, I was also facing bankruptcy. I felt ashamed, lost and out of my depth, with a brick wall in front of me every which way I turned. The critic in my head would say on repeat; "you've messed up your life. You've messed your children's lives up." I felt like my sanity was in jeopardy, and my nerves were in tatters.

The most significant part of this was my busy mind. I was so hard on myself, and I was always putting myself down. I just hated myself, as I believed my inner dialogue of failure, self-loathing and hatred. There was a real sense of guilt which would run through me as I reflected on how and why I could have brought my children into a world of chaos and misery. I believed I was a complete and utter shambolic mess, and I felt sure that I had brought it all upon myself.

The reality was; I had two options. I could allow myself to plummet further down the hole that I felt I had created (which wasn't an option, because of my children), or I find a way out of this situation. I didn't know what the answer was. I just knew that I yearned to feel free from the torture that had become my life.

Freedom to me was not living in the prison of my mind, lost in a myriad of pessimistic thoughts and crippled by intense negative emotions. All I wished for back then, was some respite from my apparent living hell. However, my immediate attention was now focused on trying to sort some basic needs out, such as food in the fridge, an income, and a home to be able to keep my children safe. I thought that if I had that, everything would be ok.

The choice seemed limited, as I crawled through daily survival mode, hour by hour. It felt like my entire body was frantically buzzing, my heart pounding, head racing, my thoughts were erratic and constant. It was like I was suffocating, with no relief or opportunity to come up for air and just breathe. From the moment

I opened my eyes, I would be keeping myself above water, treading so fast. It became like an addictive distraction, but it was so incredibly exhausting.

I could only get to sleep because I was drinking to numb my feelings. I was alcohol-reliant back then for sure. A drink would give me a moment to breathe. I needed a break from my persistently busy mind and the heaviness of my emotions. It was my easiest option since, socially, it was acceptable to go and buy a bottle of wine or two. Nobody noticed, if I'm honest. I would reason with myself, "after all, it wasn't like I was off to buy a bag of heroin!" I always knew deep within that I was escaping, but I was nowhere near being able to face that bitter truth.

Some days I would long for it to be after lunchtime, so I could open a bottle, semi-guilt free. After lunch made me less likely to question my behaviour. This lifestyle became a negative cycle, very quickly. As soon as I'd wake up sober the next day, my mind would be even busier, and the emotions would be much more damaging. They felt awful, and I was riddled with shame, fear, guilt, a total lack of self-love, and a tremendous amount of self-sabotage.

Interestingly, on the outside, people probably didn't realise what was going on inside of me. I had mastered the art of putting on a front. It became my protection blanket from people. It stopped people asking all the time, "how are you?" and "what is going on with your life?" It was the last thing I wanted. I couldn't run the risk of potentially drawing attention to myself. That would mean facing up to the fact that I wasn't coping and, even worse, I may have to address my part in all of it.

Taking personal responsibility at that time was not something I was ready to even see, let alone address. I was angry, upset, fearful and drowning in a pool of self-pity. How I distracted myself from this was by going into automatic pilot, pretending, acting and simply being busy. I got so busy my feet did not touch the ground. My ego had created a persona, and I worked hard to ensure the cracks were never revealed. I was very good at this. I was an expert at papering over the cracks. To the outside world, my ego was leading the parade. Unaware, back in my lowest times, I was addicted to being the victim. I would tell anyone who would listen to my story - the doom and gloom of my life - making sure that in all cases I started with blaming everybody else's part in the situation - other than myself. I would project continuously about what others had done or not done. What I was saying was, "I hate myself. I have created this scenario in my life, and I am a loser. I just feel that I've messed my life up."

Instead of looking inwards at my discord, I was blaming other people for what happened. I was so desperate to project the negative emotions that I was feeling, outwards. I didn't know what to do with them. I didn't realise my life was a direct reflection of what was going on for me in my subconscious mind.

I was living in survival mode, and the 3 children were so young; three, two, and six months old, which, on its own, was a full-time job. But I was also juggling a bankruptcy, a tax investigation, making a living (working) to pay for the kids and me and fighting off strangers who would turn up to my door saying that money needs to be paid. I would take costume jewellery, scarves and handbags around hair and beauty salons, put it into cabinets and sell the merchandise through the salons to make a living. For some time, I was living hand to mouth and sometimes not even making that work. I was surviving. I didn't even have enough money to have any hot water at one point. With the little bit of money I had, I would have to get the kid's food and nappies, and then the rest of it would go on wine, which, I know was not ideal, but that is how I coped.

My mind was working overtime, making everything a hundred times worse. One of the philosophies I follow today is; "deal with things as they are, not worse than they are." It is so interesting how we clump things together in our minds and make the problems overwhelming to the point, we make ourselves ill due to acute worry and obsessive thought. A friend recently said to me "you are only ever given what you can handle in life." I believe that. Though if you would have told me that when I was in the middle of that extremely challenging time, I would have had a completely different opinion.

Back then, I felt that everything was a struggle. I would go to the shop to get something, and if they didn't have it in that shop, I'd have to go somewhere else. Then the kids would be hungry or tired or need their nappies changing, and my phone would be ringing because somebody wanted some money or I would need to be at an appointment, I'd be late, everything was hard. It was all just so hard.

Then the anxiety got so bad I started to have panic attacks. I had never experienced a panic attack before. The first time it happened, I thought I was dying. I'd never seen anyone have a panic attack, so I had no clue what was happening. I thought, "Well, this is it then. I'm about to die." It was so scary. My vision went, my hearing changed, I heard what I imagined is the tone/ sound of creation, a high-pitched Om-like noise. People would talk to me, and it was like I was not there. It was like I'd checked out. Then I'd get anxious that people could tell and so I'd feel paranoid. I'd feel like I needed to run or get out of wherever I was fast. I wouldn't be able to breathe, thoughts such as, "Oh, my Gosh, I can't breathe, I can't breathe. I need to get out of here" would whizz around my head. If I was anywhere public, I'd have to bolt and get out. Life couldn't continue to be like this. It was painful, crippling and unpredictable. Life did continue this way for about a year; living inside my head, looking after my three children, trying to make enough money to feed us and doing everything I could to keep the debt collectors from the door. I was desperately searching outside myself to find the answer that would "fix" everything. Believing that I was broken. There had to be something or someone who knew how to make this better.

Previously to this, in 1999, I travelled through India with a girl who had spoken about a guy called Tony Robbins. She said that he was an incredible man and that he saved lives! That's all I could remember. I'm sure she spoke more about him, but my only memory was there's a man called Tony Robbins, and he saves people's lives.

At that moment, I needed my life saving. I thought I needed someone else to save me, though. It became apparent that the only salvation you ever need to do is your own, once I repointed my attention into a new way of being. The first step of this was taking personal responsibility for my life. So, I went to see Tony Robbins. I didn't realise it until later on. I just knew he was the only hope I had of me "being saved" at that moment.

Looking back, I recognise I was given a break, some luck, call it what you like. Luck began when I had no money, however. I was desperate to find out more about this Tony Robbins guy. I searched and searched until I found a number to call. The lady, on the other end of the phone must have thought I was a bit crackers after I gave her my list of reasons for needing to see him. She told me he was coming to London in a couple of weeks. I still had some credit cards that hadn't been cut off yet from the bankruptcy. When I got on the phone to the lady on the booking call, I knew I had to be transparent. I began by saying, "look, I'm about to lose everything in my life. I need to see this man. I've got six credit cards here; can we try them all and maybe one of them will go through. If it's meant to be, one of them will go through." And the fifth one did!

How did I know I needed to take this risk? It was an internal knowing that this is what I needed to do. I needed to go down to London and meet this man. We all have a deep, inner knowing, but we don't always listen or trust it enough. I thought that there would have only been about thirty people there, so I was slightly shocked when I realised that there were ten thousand other people there to see him too.

The moment Tony Robbins came on stage and started speaking, I was instantly blown away with what he was saying. I listened for four days solidly, I didn't dare move off my seat, I took notes, I absorbed, I spoke, I just did whatever I could. I immersed myself one hundred percent into it. It gave me such hope for the first time in a very long time. I didn't have all the answers at that point, but I had an inner flicker, like a flame that intuitively said, "I can switch my life around."

Oddly, as I observed and studied Tony Robbins, I felt a real desire to want to be doing something like this in my life. Something that meant helping others. Of course, it was laughable back then, as my own life was such a car crash. I knew that at first, I needed to make some drastic changes in my own life. The first part of changing was to focus on my inward relationship with myself. It began by implementing some of the tools I'd learnt from Tony.

He didn't teach me how to change my relationship from within, but he empowered me to start taking steps towards having "hope" and being able to find the answers to how I was going to do this. Even though I didn't know what I was searching for at that time. I had a burning desire and a magnet like experience that was guiding me. It was like an inner compass; the clearer I became, the easier it became to listen to and observe what my next intuitive move was.

After the seminar, I remember being sat on the train going home, and I had a large Tony Robbins folder that

I'd been given, it was on my knee, and a guy who sat next to me said, "Oh, have you been to a seminar?" I was radiating, oozing newfound energy. I knew it, and it was like a switch had been turned back on in me. I knew that this was the start of a new journey for me, and I knew there was a lot more to learn and to work through but it felt like I'd been given a chance.

The man sat next to me, started speaking and asking me questions about it. I felt so comfortable after those four days that I could have a conversation with somebody again, somebody that I didn't know. That's how much the light was back on. Four days before, if somebody had spoken to me, I would have just died because I was still in that anxiety, stress, survival mode, "don't look at me, don't speak to me, I'm a loser, I hate myself mode." Four days later and a new light had gone on. It wasn't entirely on, but it was enough for me to be able to feel comfortable enough to speak with a stranger on the train. That was huge.

On that journey home, I made the decision that I was going to stop smoking and stop drinking. There were a few people I needed to remove from my life, or I needed to remove myself from theirs, and that's what I did. I also made a pact to start implementing the new tools from Tony into my life straight away. Anybody who's been dependent on drinking will know it's not that easy just to go to a four-day seminar and then say, "Woohoo, I am healed." I did taper off, and I didn't always get it right. Eventually I stopped.

I also got away from certain people in my life, and that was a significant move. Tony Robbins told me that you become the four or five people that you spend most of your time with - they impact 80% to 90% of your life, and that really struck a chord with me. I started to see life like that. Asking myself questions like "where and who am I investing my time and life into? Does it serve? Is it healthy? Are these relationships empowering?" My vibration had got to such a low that I was attracting people who were like vultures in my life. I seemed to be attracting people who would take, even when I had nothing left to give. I knew that I needed to shift "ME" to shift these kind of people out of my world.

After this intense period, I put myself back in University to finish my Business Management degree. I also went on a considerable soul-searching journey. It was different back then as you didn't have access to the online platforms and resources you can now tap into free of charge. The internet was new, and all I had was an email address. There was no Facebook, YouTube or Google, so I started reading; reading everything and anything I could get my hands on. Growth, the mind, personal development, limiting beliefs, success, joy, meditation, consciousness, health, expansion, happiness, gratitude, connection, love, healing, human potential, quantum physics, metaphysics, neuroscience, motivation, energy, alternative medicine, relationships, laughter, mind body connection, truth, emotions, thoughts, you name it, I read it. The more I read, the more things started to show up. I then began attending events, talks, groups. I became a personal development junkie.

I graduated in 2006 and was quickly offered a job as a business advisor. Once I'd settled into the role, working with business start-ups, my next light bulb moment was presented. I had rapidly begun to see some everyday struggles with customers; mainly self-belief, confidence and self-worth issues. It was fascinating for me because as I started to share the little I knew, I realised that other people were also beginning to benefit from me passing on this knowledge. It felt great, I was of service, and I felt alive, fulfilled and excited to see others also transform.

It was at this point that the company came to me and said that part of their policy involved all employees doing some development work. They told me that I must do some training to learn something new and asked what I wanted to do I said, "Oh, I don't know." And they said, "Well, think about it and let us know." That weekend, like a bit of magic, low and behold, through my door, a flyer from a magazine. It was an advert for a taster weekend of how to become a life coach.

I thought, "Oh, my gosh, Tony Robbins is a life coach." My immediate thought was "I want to be like Tony, and I would love to train as a life coach."

Perhaps unsurprisingly, I went to that free weekend with The Coaching Academy U.K. It was terrific. At the end of the weekend, the inevitable happened, and they talked about the price: £4,500. My heart just sank. It was an unbelievable amount of money for me. Even though I wouldn't be paying for it, I had a gut instinct that once I went back to work and told them how much it was, that it would be a big fat no. So, I went back, and they asked me, and I told them how much it was, and it was a big fat no.

On the following Monday, I went back to my office and instantly felt inspired to write a letter to the board of the company to express my desire to do this training. So, I did. I then went to my boss. I gave her the letter, asked her to take it to the next board meeting in three days and give it to the board of directors. Her reply was sceptical, "Well, I will. But don't get your hopes up, because we've never spent more than a thousand pounds on an employee for training."

She went to the meeting, and somehow, I managed to forget about it. About a week later she came to my office, knocked on the door and just stood there and said, "I don't know how you've done it. They said yes."

I burst into tears, as I jumped up and ran toward my boss, who was quite a large capacious lady in her late sixties - she was lovely but not affectionate and regimented. I just lost it at that moment. I grabbed her and hugged her. She didn't embrace me back, but I will always be grateful for this life-changing break.

The day came that I started the training, and I flew through it all. I'd never got A's or A*s for anything, but I did with this. It was in total and utter alignment. It was almost like an angel above had made this happen. I can't explain it, and it was like that feeling when you just know something with every cell of your body is right, you know you're doing what you're meant to be doing. Previously, every cell of my body was in survival mode. Now every cell of my body was in alignment; what a contrast.

Since having this experience, one of the biggest lessons I took away is that human beings are much more powerful than we realise. The suffering that humans experience is subjective; it's an internal experience; it's happening within yourself. It seems like it's objective. Which as mentioned before means it is optional suffering. It looks like it's the outside world that is causing your suffering yet It has nothing to do with the outside world. Instead, it has everything to do with your relationship with the outside world and with yourself. Once I realised this, it gave me such a boost of self-empowerment. To realise that nothing on the outside of me can ever harm me: liberating.

During my training to become a coach, I came across the Ishaya monks through a friend. These monks have dedicated their lives to the awakening of consciousness and they're based all around the world with the head meditation centre based in Spain. I spent two and a half years learning the techniques, attending retreats and fully immersing myself in the practices before it became clear to me that the next step on my path was to train to become an Ishaya monk. I took the children out of school, and we drove to Tarragona, where we lived at the top of the Spanish mountains with the Ishayas.

Ascension, the meditation practiced by the Ishayas, taught me how to rise above the movement of the mind. With the correct meditation practise, I started to dissolve those perspectives, beliefs, and attitudes that seemingly felt real. It's not that life stops feeling real, that couldn't be further from the truth. EVERYTHING starts to feel and be experienced with much more aliveness. Living life from "here" rather than being off in my head lost in the chatter of past and future thoughts and feelings. The Bright Path Ascension taught me a different, more peaceful way.

With the Ishayas, I studied the workings of the mind and completed a programme called "Mastery of the Self" which encourages you to go inwards to dissolve limitations, stresses and negative beliefs that are stopping you from living your best life. This process is ongoing; one that I'll be on for the rest of my life. The experience has been life-changing. In 2015 I graduated, which meant that I took vows to dedicate myself to an inward journey and to then share this with the world, through teaching the Bright Path Ascension "First Sphere" courses.

This path has been about healing my relationship with myself first and continues to be. Secondly, it is about giving it all away via helping others through direct and shared experience. It is all part of the mass awakening of humanity which is taking place on our planet right now and excites me beyond belief. In my experience, learning to meditate and having my spiritual teacher, Maharishi Krishananda Ishaya, I have noticed over the past decade it's been a journey of awareness and letting life unfold rather than trying to control the outcome. Not that I always get it right; it takes continual awareness and practice.

One of the fastest ways to have the experience of being present and allowing life to unfold is through service. Service is sharing and helping others, first to become aware that they've got a choice between peace and suffering, and secondly, how to make that choice. So, for me, this book, my life, the way I live my life, is 100% dedicated back to the movement of humanity waking up.

After graduating as an Ishaya, I continued as a Life Coach. Also, I went to study the teachings of Doctor John Sarno through a SIRPA programme in the U.K. "Sarno was probably America's most famous back pain doctor. He argued that pain was the result of a psychosomatic process and emotional factors." Javier Zarracina/Vox

Dr Sarno's methodology taught me about repressed and suppressed emotions. What they are how they work in the body and how incredible the body and mind connection is. It was during this time that more and more Life Coaching clients started to arrive with physical, emotional and mental pain. All these pieces of training, combined with the observations in client's behaviours, personality, beliefs and language were resulting in me seeing patterns in pain, illness and disease. Underpinning all of this were hidden emotions such as guilt, resentment and anger which clients had unconsciously repressed into the subconscious mind.

A perfect example of this is clients presenting with Fibromyalgia. Of course, there is always going to be an exception to the rule, but 95% of the clients I've worked with suffering from Fibromyalgia have a few traits that were always prevalent. However, if I were to ask the client if they felt resentment and anger, nine times out of ten, the answer would be no. This is because it is well hidden in the subconscious; therefore, they don't necessarily feel the resentment.

The majority of clients with Fibromyalgia are usually very creative people but aren't using their creativity due to being so busy and putting everyone else first. Using your creativity and imagination isn't necessarily painting; it can be all sorts, writing, sewing, decorating etc. They are TERRIBLE at saying 'no'. They don't say 'no' because they are riddled with guilt, either consciously or unconsciously. They have learnt that taking more things on is how they believe they are accepted and loved.

As I started to see patterns in everything, I became more and more excited as I also recognised that this type of pain would change in density and often move around the body. Sometimes it may be a six-out-of-ten pain level in a specific area, the next time I saw them it would be a straight ten and be in the entire body.

As I have already mentioned, I am a prolific reader, and I came across Louise Hay about ten years ago. The first book I read was "Heal your body" which fascinated me. She mesmerised me as my eyes became opened up to the introduction and concept of the metaphysical anatomy. The best way to explain the metaphysical anatomy is that every part of the body (when in pain) is a representation of some repressed emotion and or trauma which is hidden in the subconscious mind. Louise Hay's philosophy maintains that every part of the body represents a different emotional trigger.

"You have the power to heal your life, and you need to know that. We think so often that we are helpless, but we're not. We always have the power of our minds... Claim and consciously use your power."

Heal Your Body - Louise L. Hay

It was from her research that I started reading lots about metaphysical anatomy, which led me to see the pain in a very different light. The body is reflecting a cause. I now know, through my research and experience observing and working with clients that without fail, each body part is a reflection of repressed emotions in the subconscious mind. This negative emotion wants to be freed. The more pain, the more intense the illness and disease, the more there is to let go of. The body is a road map to what's going on underneath. However, the body is so incredibly powerful that it already has everything it needs to heal.

It is from this realisation that the Freedom Alignment Method was born.

It is a method that has taken me roughly fifteen years to develop. A collaboration of the teaching that I have experienced plus observing clients with anxieties, stresses, physical, mental, emotional pain, illness and disease - and then seeing the patterns within that. It has enabled me to create a process to unravel the real truth behind the cause of a client's pain so that healing takes place and they return to health. If you would like to work with me or a member of my team privately then please book a discovery session.

www.kirsty-bortoft.com

Thank you for taking the time and effort to read through my practices, it was also my pleasure in sharing my own experiences with you.

Kirsty Bortoft - Rudra Devi Ishaya

Rudra Devi is my Ishaya name. It was given to me by spiritual teacher Maharishi Krishnananda Ishaya It is a Sanskrit name which is an ancient Vedic vibrational language which is made up of sounds rather than words. Rudra Devi means the Goddess who removes pain.

7. Bibliography

- Rudra Devi - Sanskrit Description - The Goddess that removes Pain
- Sigmund Freud - The pain/pleasure principle
- David Hawkins MD PhD - Letting Go, The Pathway to Surrender, Hay House 2nd Edition, 2014
- Evette Rose Metaphysical Anatomy - The body is talking, are you listening? Volume one, Create Space Independent Publishing Platform, Version 2, 2013
- Dr. John Sarno, The Divided Mind, Duckworth, 2008
- Dr. Bradley Nelson, The Emotion Code: How to Release Your Trapped Emotions for Abundant Health, Love, and Happiness
- Teal Swan - The Anatomy of Loneliness: How to Find Your Way Back to Connection, Watkins Publishing, New Edition, 2018
- Dr. Joe Dispenza - Summary & Analysis of Becoming Supernatural: How Common People Are Doing the Uncommon | A Guide to the Book by Dr. Joe Dispenza, Lulu.com, 2018
- Dr. Joe Dispenza - Evolve Your Brain: The Science of Changing Your Mind, Publisher Health Communications Incorporated, 2010
- Neville Goddard - Feeling is the Secret, Merchant Books, 2013

› Dr John E Sarno - The Mindbody Prescription: Healing the Body, Healing the Pain, Little, Brown and Company, First Trade Edition, 1999

› Eckhart Tolle - The Power of Now, 997 (Namaste Publishing); 1999

› Helen Schucman - A Course in Miracles, Combined Volume, Third Edition as published by the Foundation for Inner Peace. 1976 (New York: Viking: The Foundation for Inner Peace) 2007 (The Foundation for Inner Peace, 3rd ed.)

› David R Hawkins - Healing and Recovery, Hay House

› Aimee E. Raupp - Body Belief, Hay house

› Debbie Shapiro - Your Body Speaks Your Mind Decoding the Emotional, Psychological, and Spiritual Messages That Underlie Illness Book (01 Jun 2006)

› Louise Hay - You can create an extraordinary life, You Can Create an Exceptional Life, Authors Louise L. Hay, Cheryl Richardson, Edition 3, reprint Publisher Hay House, Inc, 2013

› Lisa Bourbeau - Your Body's Telling You: Love Yourself, 2nd ed. Lise Publisher: Lotus Press; 2nd edition

› Brene Brown – Power of Vulnerability: Teachings on Authenticity, Connection and Courage Publisher SOUNDS TRUE INC

- Louise L. Hay - Heal Your Body, The Mental Causes for Physical Illness and the Metaphysical Way to Overcome Them, 4th Edition, Jul 2004
- www.quotetab.com
- www.livescience.com
- www.brainyquote.com Earl Nightingale
- https://en.wikipedia.org/wiki/Kinesiology
- https://blog.iqmatrix.com/pain-pleasure-principle Sigmund Freud
- www.goodreads.com John O' Donohue
- https://www.thebrightpath.com
- https://www.sirpa.org/ SIRPA
- www.scienceandhealth.com Javier Zarracina/Vox

Printed in Great Britain
by Amazon

47409456R00109